EASY GUIDE TO

POSTPARTUM RECOVERY

A Comprehensive aid to Healing and Thriving after Childbirth

Alfred Jack

ISBN : 9798335249140

Cover design by: Art Painter Library of Congress
Control Number: 2018675309
Printed in the United States of America

TABLE OF CONTENTS

INTRODUCTION

Postpartum recovery is a journey as profound as pregnancy itself. The weeks and months following childbirth, often referred to as the "fourth trimester," are a period of significant physical, emotional, and psychological transformation. For many women, this time is filled with joy and wonder at welcoming a new life into the world. However, it is also a time of immense change, adjustment, and sometimes, challenges. The aim of this book, "Postpartum Recovery," is to provide a comprehensive guide to navigating this critical period, equipping new mothers and their families with the knowledge and tools necessary to foster a healthy and supportive recovery process.

Purpose and Scope of the Book

"Postpartum Recovery" is designed to be a practical, informative, and compassionate resource for mothers, partners, and caregivers. The postpartum period is a unique phase, marked by a multitude of experiences that vary greatly from one individual to another. Recognizing this diversity, this book addresses a wide range of topics, from immediate physical recovery to long-term health and wellness. It seeks to demystify the postpartum experience, providing clear and evidence-based information while also offering supportive advice and encouragement.

The scope of this book extends beyond mere physical recovery. It delves into the emotional and psychological aspects of postpartum life, recognizing the importance of mental health alongside physical health. Moreover, it addresses the social and relational dynamics that come into play during this time, providing guidance on nurturing relationships and building a supportive network.

Understanding Postpartum Recovery

Postpartum recovery is often overshadowed by the excitement and preparation for childbirth. While much attention is given to pregnancy and delivery, the postpartum period requires equal, if not more, care and attention. It is a time when the body heals from the incredible process of childbirth, and when new parents begin to adjust to the realities of caring for a newborn. This period can be unpredictable, and each woman's experience is unique. Factors such as the type of delivery, individual health conditions, and the presence of a support system all play crucial roles in shaping the recovery experience.

The physical changes that occur postpartum can be significant. From uterine involution to hormonal shifts, the body undergoes a series of adjustments to return to its pre-pregnancy state. These changes can manifest in various ways, including postpartum bleeding, pain, and fatigue. Understanding these changes and knowing what to expect can help women feel more in control of their recovery and reduce anxiety about the unknown.

Equally important is the emotional and psychological landscape of the postpartum period. The emotional highs and lows can be profound, ranging from the joy of bonding with a newborn to the challenges of dealing with postpartum mood disorders like the baby blues, postpartum depression, and anxiety. This book emphasizes the importance of mental health and encourages seeking help when needed. It aims to reduce the stigma associated with these conditions and promotes open conversations about mental health.

Importance of Postpartum Care

The significance of postpartum care cannot be overstated. Proper care during this period not only promotes physical healing but also supports emotional well-being and fosters positive relationships. Unfortunately, postpartum care is often neglected, with many women feeling unprepared for the realities they face after childbirth. This book seeks to fill that gap by providing comprehensive guidance on all aspects of postpartum recovery.

Postpartum care involves more than just medical check-ups. It encompasses a holistic approach to health, including nutrition, hydration, physical activity, and emotional support. It also involves understanding the specific needs and challenges that may arise, such as managing pain, breastfeeding, and dealing with sleep deprivation. By addressing these topics, this book aims to empower women to take charge of their health and recovery.

The Journey Ahead

Each chapter of "Postpartum Recovery" is dedicated to exploring a different facet of the postpartum experience. The first chapter begins with the immediate postpartum period, covering the critical first 24 hours after childbirth and the physical and emotional changes that occur. This foundational chapter sets the stage for understanding the subsequent phases of recovery.

The book then delves into the specifics of physical recovery, addressing the different experiences associated with vaginal and cesarean deliveries. It provides practical advice on managing common discomforts, promoting pelvic floor health, and understanding the body's healing process. The importance of nutrition and hydration is also highlighted, with dedicated chapters providing detailed guidance on dietary needs, breastfeeding nutrition, and the role of supplements.

Emotional and mental health are given significant attention, reflecting the crucial role they play in overall well-being. Chapters on mental health explore the spectrum of postpartum mood disorders, offering strategies for coping and emphasizing the importance of seeking help. The book also addresses the oftenoverlooked topic of postpartum relationships, offering advice on maintaining strong bonds with partners and building a supportive network of family and friends.

Physical fitness and exercise are also key components of postpartum recovery. The book provides guidelines for safely resuming physical activity, with special attention to exercises that support core and pelvic floor strength. It also explores the benefits of yoga and mindfulness practices, which can aid both physical recovery and emotional well-being.

Understanding and accepting postpartum body changes is another important aspect covered in the book. The chapters on body image and self-esteem encourage a compassionate approach to the postpartum body, promoting self-acceptance and offering practical tips for feeling comfortable and confident.

Sleep and rest are critical, yet often challenging, components of postpartum recovery. The book offers practical strategies for improving sleep quality and managing the inevitable sleep disruptions that come with caring for a newborn.

Additionally, "Postpartum Recovery" addresses potential complications that may arise during the postpartum period, such as infections, postpartum hemorrhage, and blood clots. It provides guidance on recognizing warning signs and seeking prompt medical attention.

Special considerations are also made for mothers recovering from multiple births, those who have experienced loss, and adoptive mothers, recognizing the unique challenges they may face. The book concludes with long-term health and wellness strategies, emphasizing the importance of continued selfcare and preventive health measures.

In the appendices, readers will find useful tools and resources, including a glossary of terms, sample recovery plans, and a list of contacts for additional support. These resources are designed to complement the information provided in the main chapters and offer practical tools for daily use.

A Journey of Healing and Growth

The postpartum period is not merely a time of recovery but also a time of growth and transformation. It is a journey that requires patience, compassion, and support. By providing comprehensive information and practical advice, "Postpartum Recovery" aims to be a trusted companion for new mothers as they navigate this critical phase of life.

Whether you are a first-time mother or have experienced childbirth before, this book is designed to provide valuable insights and support. It encourages a holistic approach to postpartum care, recognizing the interconnectedness of physical, emotional, and relational well-being. As you embark on this journey, remember that every experience is unique, and it is okay to seek help and take the time you need to heal and adjust.

CHAPTER 1: THE IMMEDIATE POSTPARTUM PERIOD

The First 24 Hours: What to Expect

The first 24 hours after childbirth is a time of rapid change and adjustment for both the mother and the newborn. This period, often referred to as the "golden hour" or "fourth stage of labor," is critical for initiating the recovery process and beginning the bonding experience with the baby.

For the mother: Immediately after delivery, the mother's body begins the process of returning to its pre-pregnancy state. For those who had a vaginal delivery, this includes the expulsion of the placenta and the contraction of the uterus, a process known as uterine involution. These contractions, often called "afterpains," can be uncomfortable and are typically more intense during breastfeeding due to the release of oxytocin. Women may experience significant bleeding, known as lochia, which starts as a bright red, heavy flow and gradually lightens over the coming days and weeks.

In cases of cesarean delivery, the first 24 hours involve recovery from major abdominal surgery. The mother will likely experience soreness and may have a catheter inserted to manage urinary function. Pain management is a crucial aspect of recovery, and doctors typically provide a combination of medications to manage pain and prevent infection.

For the Baby: The newborn undergoes a critical transition from the womb to the external environment. Key processes include the initiation of breathing, the regulation of body temperature, and the establishment of feeding. The baby's first cries help expand the lungs, and initial assessments, such as the Apgar score, are performed to evaluate the baby's health. Skin-to-skin contact, often encouraged immediately after birth, is vital for regulating the baby's body temperature, heart rate, and breathing, while also promoting bonding and the establishment of breastfeeding.

Breastfeeding and Bonding: The initiation of breastfeeding within the first hour of life is highly encouraged, as this period is when the baby is most alert. Colostrum, the first form of breast milk, is rich in antibodies and nutrients, providing essential protection and nourishment. Even if the baby doesn't latch perfectly, early attempts are beneficial for both the mother and baby.

Monitoring and Observation: Both mother and baby are closely monitored during this time. The mother's vital signs, such as blood pressure, heart rate, and temperature, are regularly checked to ensure stable recovery, and the baby is observed for signs of adequate breathing and feeding. Health professionals will also monitor for potential complications, such as excessive bleeding in the mother or difficulties in the baby's adaptation to life outside the womb.

Emotional and Psychological Experiences: The first 24 hours can be a whirlwind of emotions for new parents. The mother may experience a surge of euphoria, relief, and profound love, often accompanied by tears. These feelings can be interspersed with exhaustion and, in some cases, anxiety or fear, especially for first-time parents. The immediate support from healthcare professionals and family can be invaluable in providing reassurance and guidance.

Rest and Recovery: While this time is filled with excitement and new experiences, rest is crucial. The mother, having expended a great deal of physical energy during labor, needs rest to begin the healing process. Likewise, the newborn, adjusting to a new environment, will spend a significant amount of time sleeping.

In summary, the first 24 hours postpartum are a crucial period of physical recovery and emotional adjustment. It is a time for mothers to begin healing, for babies to acclimate to the outside world, and for families to start forming bonds that will continue to grow. Understanding what to expect during this period can help alleviate anxiety and ensure that both mother and baby receive the care and support they need.

Physical Changes After Childbirth

Childbirth brings about a myriad of physical changes as a woman's body transitions from pregnancy to the postpartum state. These changes, while natural, can be surprising and sometimes challenging. Understanding them can help new mothers better manage their recovery and adjust to the new normal.

Uterine Involution and Lochia: One of the most immediate and noticeable changes is uterine involution, the process by which the uterus contracts and returns to its pre-pregnancy size. This can be accompanied by afterpains, which are similar to menstrual cramps and can vary in intensity, particularly during breastfeeding due to oxytocin release. Alongside this, women experience lochia, a type of vaginal discharge that consists of blood, mucus, and uterine tissue. Lochia starts as a bright red flow, gradually transitioning to a pinkish or brownish color, and eventually becomes a yellowish or white discharge over several weeks.

Perineal and Vaginal Changes: For those who had a vaginal delivery, the perineum—the area between the vagina and the anus—may feel sore and swollen. This discomfort can be exacerbated if there were tears or an episiotomy during delivery. Stitches, if needed, typically dissolve on their own, but the area requires careful hygiene and, sometimes, pain management. Vaginal dryness and reduced vaginal tone can also occur, partly due to hormonal changes. Over time, pelvic floor exercises can help strengthen the muscles and improve these conditions.

Breast Changes: The breasts undergo significant changes as they prepare for breastfeeding. Initially, they produce colostrum, a thick yellowish fluid rich in nutrients and antibodies. A few days postpartum, the milk "comes in," causing the breasts to feel fuller, firmer, and sometimes uncomfortable—a condition known as engorgement. For some women, this can be accompanied by leaking, tenderness, and, in some cases, plugged ducts or mastitis (a breast infection). Proper breastfeeding techniques, regular feeding, and breast care are crucial for managing these changes.

Hormonal Shifts: The postpartum period is characterized by significant hormonal fluctuations. Levels of estrogen and progesterone drop rapidly after delivery, while prolactin, the hormone responsible for milk production, increases. These hormonal changes can lead to various symptoms, including night sweats, hot flashes, and mood swings. They also contribute to the shedding of hair, a common concern among new mothers. This postpartum hair loss is usually temporary, with hair growth returning to normal within a few months.

Abdominal and Pelvic Changes: The abdominal muscles, stretched and weakened during pregnancy, may take time to regain their strength. Some women experience diastasis recti, a separation of the abdominal muscles, which can cause a noticeable bulge. Gentle exercises and physical therapy can help improve muscle tone and reduce separation. The pelvic floor muscles, which support the bladder, uterus, and rectum, may also be weakened, leading to issues such as urinary incontinence. Pelvic floor exercises, also known as Kegels, are highly recommended to strengthen these muscles.

Circulatory and Metabolic Changes: After childbirth, the body gradually reduces the increased blood volume and fluid retention that occurred during pregnancy. This process can lead to increased urination and sweating as the body sheds excess fluids. Additionally, some women may experience changes in metabolism and appetite. While the initial weight loss can be significant due to the expulsion of the baby, placenta, and amniotic fluid, further gradual weight loss may continue as the body recovers and breastfeeding increases caloric needs.

Cesarean Recovery: For mothers who underwent a cesarean delivery, the recovery process includes additional considerations. The surgical incision requires proper care to prevent infection and ensure healing. Pain around the incision site, limited mobility, and restrictions on certain activities are common during the initial recovery period. It is important for these mothers to follow medical advice, manage pain effectively, and avoid heavy lifting or strenuous activity to facilitate healing.

General Well-being: Postpartum fatigue is a common experience due to the physical exertion of childbirth, hormonal changes, and the demands of caring for a newborn. Adequate rest, hydration, and a balanced diet are essential for recovery. Regular postpartum check-ups are crucial for monitoring the mother's physical health and addressing any complications that may arise.

In conclusion, the physical changes after childbirth are extensive and varied. They reflect the body's remarkable ability to adapt and recover. While some changes are temporary, others may require ongoing management and care. Understanding these changes and seeking appropriate support can help new mothers navigate the postpartum period with confidence and resilience.

Emotional and Psychological Changes

The postpartum period is not only a time of physical recovery but also a significant emotional and psychological transition. The arrival of a new baby brings about profound changes in a mother's life, and the hormonal shifts, sleep deprivation, and new responsibilities can lead to a complex array of emotions. Understanding these changes is crucial for both the mother and her support system, as they navigate this transformative phase.

The Baby Blues: One of the most common emotional experiences during the postpartum period is the "baby blues." This condition affects approximately 70-80% of new mothers and typically begins a few days after childbirth. The baby blues are characterized by mood swings, tearfulness, anxiety, and feelings of overwhelm. These symptoms are generally mild and transient, often resolving within two weeks without the need for medical intervention. The baby blues are largely attributed to the hormonal changes that occur after childbirth, including the rapid drop in estrogen and progesterone levels.

Postpartum Depression: Unlike the baby blues, postpartum depression (PPD) is a more severe and persistent mood disorder that affects around 10-20% of new mothers. PPD can occur anytime within the first year postpartum and may be influenced by a combination of hormonal, genetic, and environmental factors. Symptoms of PPD include persistent sadness, loss of interest in activities, fatigue, changes in sleep and appetite, feelings of guilt or worthlessness, and difficulty bonding with the baby. In severe cases, thoughts of harming oneself or the baby may occur. PPD requires professional treatment, which may include therapy, medication, or a combination of both. Early intervention and support are crucial for recovery.

Postpartum Anxiety: Alongside depression, postpartum anxiety is another common emotional challenge. This condition involves excessive worry or fear about the baby's health, safety, and well-being. Mothers may experience intrusive thoughts, panic attacks, and physical symptoms such as rapid heartbeat and shortness of breath. Postpartum anxiety can significantly impact a mother's quality of life and her ability to care for her baby. Like PPD, it is treatable, and seeking help from healthcare professionals is important.

Postpartum Psychosis: A rare but serious condition, postpartum psychosis affects approximately 1-2 in 1,000 women after childbirth. It typically begins within the first two weeks postpartum and is characterized by symptoms such as hallucinations, delusions, severe confusion, and disorganized thinking. Women experiencing postpartum psychosis may have difficulty distinguishing reality from their thoughts, and there is a significant risk of self-harm or harm to the baby. This condition is a medical emergency that requires immediate intervention, often involving hospitalization and treatment with antipsychotic medications.

Impact on Relationships: The postpartum period can also strain relationships. New mothers may feel a sense of isolation or frustration if their partner, family, or friends do not fully understand their experiences or provide the support they need. Open communication and shared responsibilities can help alleviate some of these challenges. Partners, in particular, play a crucial role in providing emotional and practical support, and their involvement can significantly impact the mother's well-being.

Identity and Role Adjustment: Many new mothers experience a shift in their sense of identity and selfconcept. The transition to motherhood can bring joy and fulfillment, but it can also lead to feelings of loss or confusion as women navigate their new roles. Balancing the demands of caring for a newborn with personal aspirations and previous routines can be challenging. Some women may struggle with the pressure to meet societal expectations of motherhood, which can contribute to feelings of inadequacy or self-doubt.

Coping Strategies and Support: Developing effective coping strategies is essential for managing the emotional and psychological changes during the postpartum period. These strategies can include establishing a routine, seeking support from family and friends, engaging in self-care activities, and finding time for rest. Professional support, such as therapy or counseling, can provide a safe space for mothers to explore their feelings and develop healthy coping mechanisms. Support groups, either inperson or online, can also offer valuable connections with other mothers experiencing similar challenges.

The Role of Healthcare Providers: Healthcare providers, including obstetricians, midwives, pediatricians, and mental health professionals, play a critical role in identifying and addressing postpartum emotional and psychological changes. Routine postpartum check-ups should include assessments of the mother's mental health, with an emphasis on screening for PPD, anxiety, and other mood disorders. Providing education about the signs and symptoms of these conditions, as well as available resources, can empower mothers to seek help when needed.

In summary, the emotional and psychological changes that occur after childbirth are diverse and complex. While they can be challenging, they are also a normal part of the postpartum experience. Recognizing these changes, seeking support, and accessing appropriate treatment can help new mothers navigate this period with resilience and hope. It is important to remember that experiencing emotional difficulties does not diminish a mother's ability or worth, and with the right support, recovery and a fulfilling postpartum experience are possible.

Hospital Stay vs. Home Birth Recovery

The setting in which a woman gives birth can significantly influence her postpartum recovery experience. Whether the birth occurs in a hospital, birthing center, or at home, each environment presents unique advantages and considerations. Understanding the differences can help mothers and families make informed decisions that align with their preferences and medical needs.

Hospital Birth Recovery: Hospitals are the most common setting for childbirth in many parts of the world, offering access to comprehensive medical care and facilities. For women who have high-risk pregnancies or complications during labor, hospitals provide immediate access to medical interventions, such as cesarean sections, neonatal intensive care, and advanced pain management options.

In the immediate postpartum period, hospital recovery is characterized by continuous monitoring and support from healthcare professionals. Nurses and doctors routinely check the mother's vital signs, manage pain, and provide assistance with breastfeeding and newborn care. The structured environment of a hospital can offer reassurance, especially for first-time mothers or those who have experienced complicated deliveries. The availability of lactation consultants, pediatric care, and educational resources can also be beneficial during this time.

However, the hospital setting may have some downsides. The clinical environment can feel impersonal or restrictive, with hospital policies sometimes limiting the presence of family members or dictating visiting hours. Privacy may be limited, especially in shared rooms, and the constant monitoring can disrupt rest and bonding time. Some mothers may find the hospital's schedule for examinations, meal times, and procedures intrusive.

For those who undergo cesarean deliveries, the hospital stay typically lasts longer—ranging from two to four days—compared to a vaginal delivery. This extended stay allows for monitoring of the surgical incision, pain management, and ensuring the mother is comfortable with newborn care before discharge. After discharge, follow-up visits are scheduled to monitor recovery and address any complications that may arise.

Home Birth Recovery: Home births, often facilitated by midwives, offer a more intimate and personalized birthing experience. For women with low-risk pregnancies who prefer a natural, noninterventionist approach, home births can provide a comfortable and familiar environment. The presence of family members and the freedom to move around, eat, and labor in various positions can contribute to a more relaxed and empowering experience.

Postpartum recovery at home is characterized by continuity of care. Midwives or home birth practitioners often remain with the mother for several hours after delivery to monitor the health of both mother and baby, assist with the initial stages of breastfeeding, and ensure a safe transition to the postpartum period. The comfort of being in one's own home can promote relaxation and bonding, as the new family adjusts to their new dynamic without the interruptions common in hospital settings.

A key benefit of home birth recovery is the individualized care and attention provided by the midwife or doula. They offer guidance on postpartum self-care, newborn care, and breastfeeding support, tailored to the specific needs and preferences of the mother. This personalized approach can foster a sense of confidence and control over the postpartum experience.

However, there are considerations to keep in mind with home births. The lack of immediate access to medical interventions in case of complications is a significant factor. In the event of an emergency, transfer to a hospital may be necessary, which can be stressful and time-sensitive. Additionally, home births require thorough preparation, including having the necessary supplies, a plan for postpartum care, and clear communication with a healthcare provider for follow-up care.

Hybrid Models and Birthing Centers: Some families opt for a middle ground between hospital and home births by choosing birthing centers. These centers provide a homelike environment with access to professional medical care and emergency facilities if needed. Birthing centers often emphasize natural childbirth and offer amenities such as birthing pools, comfortable rooms, and the presence of family members. They provide a more relaxed setting than hospitals while maintaining a higher level of medical oversight than a home birth.

Postpartum Care Considerations: Regardless of the birth setting, the postpartum period requires careful attention to the physical and emotional needs of the mother. Key considerations include managing pain, monitoring for signs of infection or complications, supporting breastfeeding, and addressing emotional well-being. For home births, having a plan for follow-up care with a healthcare provider is crucial to ensure both mother and baby are healthy.

CHAPTER 2: PHYSICAL RECOVERY

Healing After Vaginal Delivery

Healing after a vaginal delivery is a multifaceted process that involves several physical and emotional aspects. The body undergoes significant changes during childbirth, and the recovery process is essential for restoring health and well-being. While each woman's experience is unique, understanding the common elements of recovery can help new mothers navigate this period with greater ease and confidence. **Perineal Healing:** The perineum, the area between the vagina and anus, often undergoes significant stretching and, in some cases, tearing during vaginal delivery. Perineal tears or episiotomies (surgical cuts made to enlarge the vaginal opening) can vary in severity from minor first-degree tears to more extensive third or fourth-degree tears. The healing process for these injuries can take several weeks and involves managing pain, preventing infection, and promoting tissue repair. Ice packs, sitz baths, and over-thecounter pain relief medications are commonly recommended to alleviate discomfort. Proper hygiene, including regular washing with mild soap and water, is crucial to prevent infection. For more severe tears, follow-up with a healthcare provider is important to ensure proper healing.

Uterine Involution: After delivery, the uterus begins the process of returning to its pre-pregnancy size, a process known as uterine involution. This process involves the contraction of the uterine muscles, which can cause cramping known as afterpains. These cramps may be more pronounced during breastfeeding due to the release of oxytocin, which stimulates uterine contractions. While afterpains can be uncomfortable, they are a normal part of the healing process and typically diminish within a few days. Maintaining adequate hydration and using pain relief medications, if needed, can help manage discomfort.

Vaginal Discharge (Lochia): Lochia, the vaginal discharge that occurs after childbirth, is another aspect of postpartum recovery. This discharge consists of blood, mucus, and uterine tissue and goes through several stages. Initially, lochia is bright red and heavy, resembling a heavy menstrual period. Over the following weeks, it gradually becomes lighter in color and volume, transitioning from red to pink, brown, and finally yellow or white. The duration of lochia varies, but it typically lasts four to six weeks. It's important for mothers to monitor the flow and color of lochia, as heavy bleeding or a sudden increase in flow can indicate a complication and should be reported to a healthcare provider.

Physical Rest and Activity: Rest is crucial in the initial stages of postpartum recovery. The body requires time to heal from the physical exertion of childbirth, and new mothers should prioritize rest and avoid strenuous activities. However, gentle movement and light exercises, such as walking, can promote circulation and aid in recovery. Gradually increasing activity levels, as tolerated, is recommended. Pelvic floor exercises, or Kegel exercises, can help strengthen the pelvic floor muscles, which may have been stretched or weakened during childbirth.

Emotional Well-being: The emotional aspect of healing after vaginal delivery is also important. New mothers may experience a range of emotions, from joy and relief to anxiety and fatigue. It's essential to acknowledge these feelings and seek support from family, friends, or healthcare providers as needed. Postpartum blues, characterized by mood swings, tearfulness, and irritability, are common and typically resolve within two weeks. However, if these symptoms persist or worsen, it may be indicative of postpartum depression, and professional help should be sought.

Nutrition and Hydration: Proper nutrition and hydration play a key role in the healing process. A balanced diet rich in nutrients supports tissue repair and energy levels. Staying hydrated is particularly important, especially for breastfeeding mothers, as it aids in milk production and overall well-being. In conclusion, healing after a vaginal delivery involves a combination of physical recovery, emotional adjustment, and self-care. By understanding the common aspects of this process and following recommended care practices, new mothers can support their recovery and transition into parenthood more smoothly.

Healing After Cesarean Section

Cesarean section (C-section) is a major surgical procedure that requires a unique recovery process distinct from vaginal delivery. Healing after a C-section involves not only recovering from childbirth but also managing the surgical incision and the associated physical and emotional challenges. Understanding the specific aspects of C-section recovery can help new mothers navigate this period with greater awareness and preparedness.

Incision Care: One of the primary concerns after a C-section is the care of the surgical incision. The incision is typically made horizontally just above the pubic hairline, though in some cases, it may be vertical. Proper care of the incision site is crucial to prevent infection and promote healing. This includes keeping the area clean and dry, avoiding tight clothing that may irritate the incision, and monitoring for signs of infection such as redness, swelling, or unusual discharge. Healthcare providers often provide specific instructions for incision care, including when and how to remove any surgical dressings and how to clean the area. Stitches, staples, or surgical glue may be used to close the incision, and the method used will determine the specific care needed.

Pain Management: Pain management is a significant aspect of C-section recovery. The surgery involves cutting through skin, fat, and muscle layers, which can result in considerable discomfort during the initial recovery period. Pain relief options may include prescription medications, over-the-counter pain relievers, and non-pharmacological methods such as heat packs or gentle movement. It is important for mothers to follow their healthcare provider's recommendations for pain management, as adequate pain control can improve mobility and overall recovery. However, caution is advised with medications, especially for breastfeeding mothers, to ensure they are safe for both the mother and the baby.

Mobility and Activity: While rest is crucial after a C-section, early mobilization is also encouraged to promote circulation and reduce the risk of complications such as blood clots. New mothers are often encouraged to start walking as soon as they feel able, even if it is just a short distance. Gradually increasing the level of activity is beneficial, but it is important to avoid heavy lifting, strenuous exercise, or any activity that puts strain on the abdominal muscles until fully healed. This typically means refraining from such activities for at least six weeks, though this can vary based on individual recovery.

Postpartum Symptoms: In addition to managing the surgical incision, mothers recovering from a Csection experience typical postpartum symptoms such as lochia, afterpains, and breastfeeding challenges. Lochia is generally lighter in women who have had a C-section compared to those who delivered vaginally, but it still goes through similar stages. Afterpains, caused by uterine contractions as the uterus returns to its pre-pregnancy size, may also occur, though they are usually less intense. Breastfeeding can present unique challenges after a C-section, particularly if the surgery was unplanned or if the mother is experiencing significant pain. However, many women successfully breastfeed after a C-section, and lactation consultants can provide valuable support and guidance.

Emotional Recovery: The emotional aspect of recovering from a C-section is also significant. Women may experience a range of emotions, from relief and joy to disappointment or frustration, particularly if the C-section was unplanned or differed from their birth plan. The physical limitations and longer recovery time can also be challenging, especially when combined with the demands of caring for a newborn. It's important for mothers to seek emotional support from partners, family, friends, or mental health professionals if needed. Postpartum depression and anxiety are risks for all new mothers, regardless of the type of delivery, and it is crucial to recognize and address these conditions early.

Follow-Up Care: Regular follow-up care is essential after a C-section. This includes visits to a healthcare provider to check on the healing of the incision, monitor for complications, and discuss any concerns the mother may have. These appointments are also an opportunity to receive guidance on resuming physical activities, contraception options, and overall health and well-being.

In conclusion, healing after a C-section involves careful attention to incision care, pain management, and gradual return to activity. Emotional support and follow-up care are equally important to ensure a smooth recovery. With proper care and support, most women recover fully and can successfully transition into their new roles as mothers.

Managing Pain and Discomfort

Managing pain and discomfort is a crucial aspect of postpartum recovery, as the body undergoes significant changes and adjustments after childbirth. Whether the delivery was vaginal or via cesarean section, new mothers often experience a range of discomforts, including pain from the delivery process, uterine contractions, breastfeeding challenges, and general soreness. Effective pain management strategies can help alleviate discomfort, promote healing, and improve the overall postpartum experience.

Postpartum Pain Sources: The sources of postpartum pain and discomfort are varied and can include:

1. **Perineal Pain:** For women who have had a vaginal delivery, perineal pain can result from tearing, episiotomy, or general stretching during childbirth. This pain may be accompanied by swelling and bruising in the perineal area.

2. **Cesarean Incision Pain:** Mothers who have undergone a cesarean section may experience pain at the incision site. This can include sharp, stabbing pain, tenderness, and sensitivity around the surgical area.

3. **Uterine Contractions (Afterpains):** As the uterus contracts to return to its pre-pregnancy size, women may experience afterpains. These contractions can be particularly noticeable during breastfeeding due to the release of oxytocin.

4. **Breast Engorgement:** Breastfeeding mothers may experience breast engorgement, which can cause significant discomfort, especially during the early days of breastfeeding.

5. **Muscle Aches and Joint Pain:** The physical exertion of labor, combined with changes in posture and the physical demands of caring for a newborn, can lead to muscle aches and joint pain.

Pain Management Strategies:

1. **Medications:** Pain relief medications, both over-the-counter and prescription, are commonly used to manage postpartum pain. Nonsteroidal anti-inflammatory drugs (NSAIDs) like ibuprofen can be effective for reducing pain and inflammation. For more severe pain, especially after a cesarean section, doctors may prescribe stronger pain medications. It's important for breastfeeding mothers to consult with their healthcare provider to ensure that any medications taken are safe for the baby.

2. **Cold and Heat Therapy:** Cold packs can be applied to the perineal area or incision site to reduce swelling and numb the area, providing relief from pain. Sitz baths, which involve sitting in warm

water, can also soothe perineal pain and promote healing. Heat packs can help relax sore muscles and alleviate cramping.

3. **Rest and Positioning:** Adequate rest is essential for postpartum recovery. Finding comfortable positions for sitting and lying down can help alleviate discomfort, especially for those recovering from a cesarean section. Using pillows to support the abdomen, back, and breasts can also reduce strain and improve comfort.

4. **Pelvic Floor Exercises:** Kegel exercises can help strengthen the pelvic floor muscles, which may have been stretched or weakened during childbirth. These exercises can alleviate pain and discomfort associated with perineal trauma and help prevent issues like urinary incontinence.

5. **Breast Care:** For breastfeeding mothers, proper breast care is important to prevent and manage engorgement, blocked ducts, and mastitis. Regular breastfeeding or pumping, warm compresses, and gentle breast massage can help relieve engorgement and prevent complications.

6. **Emotional Support:** Emotional well-being is closely linked to physical pain perception. New mothers may experience heightened sensitivity to pain if they are feeling anxious, overwhelmed, or stressed. Emotional support from partners, family, friends, or mental health professionals can provide comfort and reduce the perception of pain.

7. **Professional Support:** Healthcare providers, including obstetricians, midwives, and lactation consultants, can offer valuable guidance and support in managing postpartum pain. They can provide specific recommendations based on the type of delivery, the presence of any complications, and the mother's overall health.

8. **Alternative Therapies:** Some women find relief from postpartum pain through alternative therapies such as acupuncture, chiropractic care, or herbal remedies. It's important to discuss any alternative therapies with a healthcare provider to ensure they are safe and appropriate.

Monitoring and Communication: It is essential for new mothers to monitor their pain levels and communicate with their healthcare providers about any concerns. Persistent or severe pain, unusual symptoms, or signs of infection should be reported promptly, as they may indicate complications that require medical attention.

Pelvic Floor Health and Rehabilitation

Pelvic floor health is a critical component of postpartum recovery, as the muscles and tissues of the pelvic floor undergo significant strain during pregnancy and childbirth. The pelvic floor supports the pelvic organs, including the bladder, uterus, and rectum, and plays a crucial role in urinary and fecal continence, sexual function, and overall core stability. After childbirth, especially after vaginal delivery, many women experience issues such as pelvic organ prolapse, urinary incontinence, and weakened pelvic floor muscles. Rehabilitation of the pelvic floor is essential for restoring strength and function, and it can have a profound impact on a woman's quality of life.

Pelvic Floor Changes During Pregnancy and Childbirth: During pregnancy, the growing uterus places additional pressure on the pelvic floor muscles, causing them to stretch and weaken. Hormonal changes also play a role in relaxing the connective tissues of the pelvic floor, making them more susceptible to strain. Childbirth, particularly vaginal delivery, can further stretch and damage these muscles, especially if there are complications such as perineal tears, episiotomies, or the use of forceps or vacuum extraction. Even women who have had a cesarean section may experience pelvic floor dysfunction due to the effects of pregnancy on the pelvic region.

Common Postpartum Pelvic Floor Issues:

1. **Urinary Incontinence:** This is a common issue postpartum, characterized by the involuntary leakage of urine. Stress incontinence, which occurs during activities that increase intra-abdominal pressure (such as coughing, sneezing, or lifting), is particularly common. It is often a result of weakened pelvic floor muscles.

2. **Pelvic Organ Prolapse:** This condition occurs when the pelvic organs (such as the bladder, uterus, or rectum) descend into or outside of the vaginal canal due to weakened support structures. Symptoms can include a feeling of heaviness or pressure in the pelvic area, a bulge in the vagina, and discomfort during intercourse.

3. **Pain and Discomfort:** Some women experience pain in the pelvic region, lower back, or hips due to the strain on the pelvic floor muscles. Pain during sexual intercourse (dyspareunia) can also occur if the pelvic floor muscles are tense or if there is scar tissue from tears or episiotomy.

Rehabilitation and Strengthening:

1. **Kegel Exercises:** Kegel exercises are one of the most commonly recommended methods for strengthening the pelvic floor muscles. These exercises involve contracting and relaxing the muscles that support the pelvic organs. To perform a Kegel exercise, a woman should identify the

correct muscles by trying to stop the flow of urine. Once identified, she should contract these muscles for a few seconds and then relax, repeating the process several times. Consistent practice of Kegel exercises can improve muscle strength and reduce symptoms of incontinence and prolapse.

2. **Physical Therapy:** Pelvic floor physical therapy can be highly beneficial for postpartum women experiencing pelvic floor dysfunction. A specialized physical therapist can assess the condition of the pelvic floor muscles and provide individualized exercises and treatments. This may include biofeedback, manual therapy, and education on proper posture and body mechanics to support the pelvic floor.

3. **Core Strengthening:** Strengthening the core muscles, including the abdominal and back muscles, is important for overall pelvic stability. Gentle exercises such as pelvic tilts, bridges, and gentle abdominal exercises can help strengthen these muscles without putting excessive strain on the pelvic floor.

4. **Lifestyle Modifications:** Certain lifestyle changes can also support pelvic floor health. These may include maintaining a healthy weight, avoiding heavy lifting, practicing good posture, and managing constipation to avoid straining during bowel movements.

5. **Supportive Devices:** In some cases, healthcare providers may recommend the use of supportive devices, such as pessaries, to help support the pelvic organs and alleviate symptoms of prolapse. Pessaries are removable devices inserted into the vagina to provide support.

6. **Emotional Support:** The emotional impact of pelvic floor issues can be significant, affecting a woman's self-esteem and quality of life. It is important for women to seek emotional support and counseling if needed, and to communicate openly with healthcare providers about their symptoms and concerns.

Prevention and Long-Term Care: Maintaining pelvic floor health is a lifelong commitment. Women are encouraged to continue pelvic floor exercises and be mindful of activities that may strain these muscles, such as high-impact sports or heavy lifting. Regular check-ups with a healthcare provider can help monitor pelvic floor health and address any emerging issues.

In conclusion, pelvic floor health and rehabilitation are crucial aspects of postpartum recovery. By addressing pelvic floor dysfunction through targeted exercises, physical therapy, and lifestyle modifications, women can regain strength and function, improve their quality of life, and prevent longterm complications.

Postpartum Bleeding and Discharge (Lochia)

Postpartum bleeding and discharge, collectively known as lochia, are normal parts of the postpartum recovery process. Lochia consists of blood, mucus, and uterine tissue that is expelled from the uterus after childbirth as the body sheds the lining that supported the pregnancy. Understanding the stages of lochia, as well as the signs of normal versus abnormal bleeding, can help new mothers manage this aspect of recovery with confidence and awareness.

Stages of Lochia:

1. **Lochia Rubra:** This is the first stage of lochia, occurring during the first few days after childbirth. Lochia rubra is characterized by a bright red, heavy flow, similar to a menstrual period. It contains a significant amount of blood, along with small clots, and may have a fleshy odor. During this stage, it is normal for women to experience a heavier flow, especially when standing up after lying down, as blood may pool in the vagina while lying down.

2. **Lochia Serosa:** This stage typically begins around the fourth day postpartum and can last until about the tenth day. Lochia serosa is lighter in color, ranging from pink to brownish. The flow becomes less heavy, and the consistency changes, with a decrease in blood content and an increase in mucus and leukocytes (white blood cells). This stage indicates that the uterus is healing and the volume of discharge is gradually decreasing.

3. **Lochia Alba:** The final stage of lochia is lochia alba, which can last from the second to the sixth week postpartum. During this stage, the discharge becomes white or yellowish-white and is composed mainly of mucus and leukocytes. The flow is much lighter, and the consistency is more like that of regular vaginal discharge. Lochia alba marks the end of the uterine healing process, and the discharge gradually tapers off until it stops completely.

Managing Lochia:

1. **Hygiene:** Good hygiene is essential during the postpartum period to prevent infection. Women should use sanitary pads, not tampons, to manage the flow of lochia, as tampons can introduce bacteria into the vagina and increase the risk of infection. It is important to change pads frequently and wash the perineal area with mild soap and water. Some women may also find it helpful to use peri bottles (squirt bottles) to gently clean the area with water after using the toilet.

2. **Activity and Rest:** Physical activity can affect the flow of lochia. Increased activity, such as walking or lifting, may cause a temporary increase in bleeding. Women are advised to rest and

avoid strenuous activities during the early postpartum period to allow the body to heal. Gradually increasing activity levels, based on individual recovery, is generally recommended.

3. **Monitoring for Abnormalities:** While lochia is a normal part of postpartum recovery, it is important to be aware of signs that may indicate complications. Abnormal signs include:

o Heavy Bleeding: Soaking through a pad in less than an hour or passing large clots (larger than a golf ball) may indicate excessive bleeding and should be reported to a healthcare provider immediately.

o Foul Odor: A foul-smelling discharge may indicate an infection and should be evaluated by a healthcare provider. o Fever or Chills: These symptoms, along with abdominal pain or tenderness, may suggest an infection and require prompt medical attention.

o Sudden Increase in Bleeding: A sudden increase in bleeding after it has slowed down may indicate a problem, such as retained placental tissue or uterine atony (inability of the uterus to contract properly).

Emotional and Physical Well-being: The experience of lochia can also affect a woman's emotional and physical well-being. Some women may feel self-conscious or uncomfortable with the discharge, while others may experience relief as it signifies the body's return to a non-pregnant state. It is important for women to give themselves grace during this period and to seek support from partners, family, or healthcare providers if needed.

Postpartum Care and Follow-Up: Follow-up care is crucial for monitoring the postpartum healing process. Most women have a postpartum check-up with their healthcare provider about six weeks after delivery. During this visit, the healthcare provider will assess the healing of the uterus, check for any complications, and discuss family planning, contraception, and any other concerns the mother may have.

In summary, postpartum bleeding and discharge (lochia) are normal and expected parts of recovery after childbirth. By understanding the stages of lochia, practicing good hygiene, and being aware of signs of complications, women can manage this aspect of postpartum recovery effectively. Open communication with healthcare providers and emotional support are also key components of a positive recovery experience.

Managing Postpartum Swelling and Engorgement

Postpartum swelling and engorgement are common experiences for new mothers as their bodies adjust after childbirth. Swelling can occur in various parts of the body, including the legs, feet, and hands, due to the body's natural retention of fluids and hormonal changes. Breast engorgement, on the other hand, is a specific condition related to breastfeeding, characterized by the swelling and fullness of the breasts as they begin to produce milk. Understanding the causes, management strategies, and when to seek medical help can help women navigate these uncomfortable symptoms during the postpartum period.

Postpartum Swelling:

Causes: Swelling, also known as edema, is caused by the accumulation of excess fluid in the body's tissues. During pregnancy, the body produces extra blood and fluids to support the growing fetus, which can contribute to swelling. Additionally, hormonal changes can cause fluid retention. After childbirth, the body gradually eliminates this excess fluid, but it can take time, leading to postpartum swelling.

Common Areas of Swelling: Swelling is most commonly observed in the legs, ankles, feet, and hands. Some women may also experience swelling in the face and around the eyes. The swelling is usually more noticeable in the first few days postpartum and can be exacerbated by standing for long periods, warm weather, or high sodium intake.

Management Strategies for postpartum swelling:

1. **Rest and Elevation:** Resting and elevating the swollen limbs can help reduce swelling. Women are encouraged to prop their feet up on a pillow when sitting or lying down. Elevating the legs above heart level can help improve circulation and reduce fluid buildup.

2. **Hydration:** Drinking plenty of water can help flush excess fluids from the body. While it may seem counterintuitive, staying well-hydrated can actually reduce fluid retention.

3. Balanced Diet: A diet low in sodium can help reduce swelling by preventing fluid retention. Eating a balanced diet rich in fruits, vegetables, and lean proteins can also support overall recovery and well-being.

4. **Compression:** Wearing compression stockings or socks can help reduce swelling in the legs and improve circulation. These garments provide gentle pressure that helps prevent fluid from pooling in the lower extremities.

5. **Gentle Exercise:** Light physical activity, such as walking, can help improve circulation and reduce swelling. It is important to start with gentle exercises and gradually increase activity levels as tolerated.

6. **Cold Compresses:** Applying cold compresses to swollen areas can help reduce inflammation and discomfort.

When to Seek Medical Help: While postpartum swelling is generally normal and resolves on its own, it is important to seek medical attention if the swelling is accompanied by severe pain, redness, or warmth, as these could be signs of a blood clot. Additionally, sudden or excessive swelling, particularly in the face or hands, could indicate preeclampsia, a serious condition that requires immediate medical attention.

Breast Engorgement:

Causes: Breast engorgement occurs when the breasts become overly full of milk, blood, and lymphatic fluid. This typically happens when the milk "comes in" a few days after childbirth, but it can also occur at any time during breastfeeding if the breasts are not adequately emptied. Engorgement can be caused by infrequent feedings, poor latch, or a sudden decrease in breastfeeding or pumping.

Symptoms: Engorged breasts are swollen, firm, and often painful. They may feel warm to the touch, and the skin may appear tight and shiny. Some women also experience a low-grade fever. Engorgement can make it difficult for the baby to latch onto the breast, further complicating breastfeeding.

Management Strategies for breast feeding:

1. **Frequent Breastfeeding or Pumping:** The most effective way to relieve engorgement is to frequently breastfeed or pump to empty the breasts. This helps reduce the buildup of milk and alleviates pressure and discomfort. Ensuring a good latch is important for effective milk removal.

2. **Warm Compresses and Showers:** Applying warm compresses or taking a warm shower before breastfeeding can help stimulate milk flow and make it easier for the baby to latch. The warmth can also help relax the milk ducts and relieve some of the discomfort.

3. **Cold Compresses:** After breastfeeding or pumping, applying cold compresses to the breasts can help reduce swelling and numb the area, providing relief from pain.

4. **Hand Expression:** If the breasts are too engorged for the baby to latch, hand expression can help soften the breast tissue and make latching easier. Gently massaging the breasts can also help release milk and relieve pressure.

5. **Proper Bra Fit:** Wearing a supportive, well-fitting bra can help reduce discomfort. However, it is important to avoid bras that are too tight, as they can restrict milk flow and worsen engorgement.

6. **Pain Relief:** Over-the-counter pain relievers, such as ibuprofen, can help alleviate pain and reduce inflammation. It is important to consult a healthcare provider before taking any medications, especially if breastfeeding.

When to Seek Medical Help: If engorgement is not relieved by breastfeeding or pumping, or if there are signs of infection such as redness, warmth, severe pain, or fever, it is important to seek medical attention. These symptoms could indicate mastitis, an infection of the breast tissue that requires prompt treatment.

CHAPTER 3: EMOTIONAL AND MENTAL HEALTH

The Baby Blues vs. Postpartum Depression

The postpartum period is a time of immense change, both physically and emotionally. Many new mothers experience a range of emotions, from joy and excitement to anxiety and sadness. Two of the most common emotional experiences during this time are the "baby blues" and postpartum depression, both of which can significantly impact a mother's well-being.

The Baby Blues: The baby blues are a mild, transient emotional state that affects a majority of new mothers. Typically beginning within the first few days after childbirth, the baby blues are characterized by mood swings, tearfulness, irritability, and feelings of overwhelm. These symptoms are usually mild and peak around the fourth or fifth day postpartum, lasting for about two weeks. The baby blues are thought to result from a combination of hormonal changes, exhaustion, and the emotional adjustment to motherhood. During pregnancy, levels of estrogen and progesterone are high, and after delivery, they drop rapidly. This hormonal shift, along with the physical and emotional demands of caring for a newborn, can trigger the baby blues.

Postpartum Depression (PPD): Unlike the baby blues, postpartum depression is a more serious and prolonged condition. It can begin anytime within the first year after childbirth, though it often starts within the first few weeks. PPD is characterized by more severe symptoms, including persistent sadness, hopelessness, feelings of worthlessness, loss of interest in activities, changes in appetite and sleep patterns, fatigue, difficulty bonding with the baby, and thoughts of harming oneself or the baby. These symptoms can interfere with a mother's ability to care for herself and her child.

The exact cause of PPD is not fully understood, but it is believed to result from a combination of hormonal changes, psychological factors, and life circumstances. Risk factors for PPD include a history of depression or anxiety, lack of social support, stressful life events, and complications during pregnancy or delivery.

Differences and Similarities: While both the baby blues and PPD involve emotional disturbances, the key differences lie in the severity, duration, and impact of symptoms. The baby blues are generally mild, transient, and do not impair daily functioning, whereas PPD is more intense, long-lasting, and can significantly affect a mother's ability to function and care for her baby.

It is important to note that experiencing the baby blues does not necessarily mean a woman will develop PPD. However, it is crucial for new mothers and their families to be aware of the signs and symptoms of PPD so that appropriate support and treatment can be sought if needed.

Treatment and Support: For the baby blues, supportive care, rest, and understanding from family and friends are often sufficient to help mothers cope. For PPD, however, professional treatment is usually necessary. This may include therapy, medication, and support groups. Early intervention is important, as untreated PPD can have long-term effects on both the mother and her child, including difficulties in bonding and attachment, as well as developmental delays in the child.

In summary, while the baby blues and postpartum depression share some similarities, they are distinct conditions with different implications for a mother's emotional well-being. Recognizing the differences and seeking appropriate support can make a significant difference in a mother's recovery and overall mental health.

Anxiety and Postpartum Psychosis

In addition to depression, new mothers may experience other mental health challenges, including postpartum anxiety and, in rare cases, postpartum psychosis. These conditions can be distressing and require appropriate care and attention.

Postpartum Anxiety: Postpartum anxiety is characterized by excessive worry, fear, and nervousness that occur after childbirth. Unlike the more commonly discussed postpartum depression, anxiety disorders in the postpartum period are less recognized but can be equally debilitating. Symptoms of postpartum anxiety may include constant worry about the baby's health and safety, fear of being alone with the baby, racing thoughts, difficulty sleeping, physical symptoms like palpitations or shortness of breath, and an overwhelming sense of dread.

Postpartum anxiety can take several forms, including generalized anxiety disorder (GAD), panic disorder, and obsessive-compulsive disorder (OCD). GAD involves pervasive worry about a variety of topics, while panic disorder is characterized by sudden, intense episodes of fear (panic attacks). Postpartum OCD may involve intrusive thoughts or fears about harming the baby, accompanied by compulsive behaviors to prevent harm.

The causes of postpartum anxiety are multifactorial and may include hormonal changes, sleep deprivation, personal or family history of anxiety disorders, and stressful life events. Women who experience high levels of anxiety during pregnancy are also at increased risk of postpartum anxiety.

Postpartum Psychosis: Postpartum psychosis is a rare but severe mental health condition that can occur suddenly after childbirth. It is considered a psychiatric emergency and requires immediate medical intervention. Symptoms typically appear within the first two weeks postpartum and may include hallucinations (seeing or hearing things that are not there), delusions (false beliefs), extreme mood swings, confusion, disorganized thinking, and behaviors that are out of character. Mothers with postpartum psychosis may have thoughts of harming themselves or their baby.

The exact cause of postpartum psychosis is not well understood, but it is believed to involve a combination of genetic, hormonal, and environmental factors. Women with a personal or family history of bipolar disorder or previous episodes of psychosis are at higher risk. Postpartum psychosis requires urgent treatment, often including hospitalization, medication, and therapy. Early intervention is crucial for the safety of both the mother and her baby.

Managing and Seeking Help: For postpartum anxiety, treatment options may include therapy, medication, and support groups. Cognitive-behavioral therapy (CBT) is particularly effective in addressing the thought patterns and behaviors associated with anxiety. Medications, such as selective serotonin reuptake inhibitors (SSRIs), may also be prescribed, especially if anxiety symptoms are severe. For postpartum psychosis, treatment usually involves antipsychotic medications and mood stabilizers. Hospitalization may be necessary to ensure the safety of the mother and baby. Ongoing support and monitoring are crucial, as postpartum psychosis can be a recurring condition.

Support and Recovery: Recovery from postpartum anxiety and psychosis is possible with appropriate treatment and support. It's important for women to communicate openly with healthcare providers about their symptoms and seek help as soon as possible. Support from partners, family, and friends can also play a vital role in the recovery process.

In summary, postpartum anxiety and psychosis are serious mental health conditions that can occur after childbirth. While postpartum anxiety is more common and can vary in severity, postpartum psychosis is a rare and severe condition that requires immediate medical attention. Early recognition and intervention are key to ensuring the well-being of the mother and her family.

Coping Strategies and When to Seek Help

The postpartum period is a time of significant adjustment, and many new mothers experience a range of emotional and mental health challenges. While it is normal to feel overwhelmed, anxious, or even sad at times, it is essential to have coping strategies in place and to know when to seek professional help.

Coping Strategies:

1. **Rest and Self-Care**: Prioritizing rest and self-care is crucial for postpartum recovery. New mothers often struggle with sleep deprivation, which can exacerbate feelings of anxiety and depression. Whenever possible, new mothers should rest when the baby sleeps and accept help from family

and friends for household chores and baby care. Engaging in self-care activities, such as taking a warm bath, reading a book, or practicing mindfulness, can also help reduce stress.

2. **Healthy Diet and Hydration**: Proper nutrition and hydration play a vital role in overall wellbeing. A balanced diet rich in fruits, vegetables, lean proteins, and whole grains can help stabilize mood and energy levels. Staying hydrated is also important, especially for breastfeeding mothers.

3. **Physical Activity**: Gentle physical activity, such as walking or postpartum yoga, can improve mood and reduce stress. Exercise releases endorphins, which are natural mood lifters. However, it is important to consult a healthcare provider before starting any exercise routine, especially after a cesarean section or complicated delivery.

4. **Support System**: Building a strong support system is essential. New mothers should reach out to family, friends, or support groups for emotional and practical support. Talking to other mothers who have gone through similar experiences can provide comfort and reduce feelings of isolation.

5. **Mindfulness and Relaxation Techniques**: Mindfulness practices, such as deep breathing, meditation, and progressive muscle relaxation, can help manage anxiety and promote relaxation. These techniques can be especially helpful during moments of stress or when feeling overwhelmed.

6. **Setting Realistic Expectations**: New mothers often put pressure on themselves to be perfect, which can lead to feelings of inadequacy. It is important to set realistic expectations and understand that it is normal to have ups and downs. Accepting that it is okay to make mistakes and that not everything will go according to plan can alleviate unnecessary stress.

7. **Journaling**: Writing down thoughts and feelings in a journal can be a therapeutic way to process emotions. Journaling allows mothers to reflect on their experiences, track their emotional journey, and identify patterns that may need attention.

When to Seek Help:

While many new mothers experience normal emotional fluctuations, there are times when professional help is necessary. It is important to seek help if:

1. **Persistent Symptoms**: If feelings of sadness, anxiety, or irritability persist for more than two weeks and do not improve, it may be a sign of a more serious condition, such as postpartum depression or anxiety.

2. **Impairment in Functioning**: If emotional symptoms interfere with daily functioning, such as the inability to care for the baby, manage household responsibilities, or maintain personal hygiene, it is crucial to seek help.

3. **Thoughts of Harm**: Any thoughts of self-harm or harming the baby are serious and require immediate medical attention. These thoughts can be a symptom of postpartum depression, anxiety, or psychosis, and it is important to seek emergency care.

4. **Physical Symptoms**: If emotional distress is accompanied by physical symptoms, such as chest pain, difficulty breathing, or dizziness, it is important to consult a healthcare provider.

5. **Lack of Interest**: A lack of interest in activities that were previously enjoyable, including bonding with the baby, can be a sign of postpartum depression and should be addressed.

The Role of Partners and Family in Emotional Support

The postpartum period can be a challenging time for new mothers, and the support of partners and family members plays a crucial role in their emotional and mental well-being. The transition to parenthood involves significant adjustments, and having a strong support system can make a substantial difference in a mother's experience and recovery.

Emotional Support from Partners:

Partners are often the primary source of emotional support for new mothers. Their involvement and understanding can significantly impact a mother's emotional health. Key aspects of a supportive partner include:

1. **Active Listening**: Partners can provide valuable support by actively listening to the mother's concerns, fears, and experiences. This involves being present, showing empathy, and validating her feelings. Avoiding judgment or offering unsolicited advice allows the mother to express herself freely.

2. **Sharing Responsibilities**: The physical and emotional demands of caring for a newborn can be overwhelming. Partners can help alleviate some of this burden by sharing responsibilities, such as feeding, diaper changes, and household chores. This not only provides practical support but also allows the mother to rest and recover.

3. **Encouragement and Reassurance**: New mothers often doubt their abilities and worry about their parenting skills. Partners can offer encouragement and reassurance, reminding them that they are doing a good job and that it is normal to have uncertainties. Positive affirmations can boost a mother's confidence and self-esteem.

4. **Monitoring for Signs of Distress**: Partners should be attentive to changes in the mother's mood and behavior. If signs of postpartum depression, anxiety, or other mental health concerns arise, partners should encourage seeking professional help. It is important to approach this conversation with sensitivity and care.

5. **Supporting Bonding**: Partners can play a role in fostering the mother-baby bond by creating opportunities for positive interactions. This can include helping with breastfeeding, facilitating skin-to-skin contact, or simply spending quality time together as a family.

The Role of Family Members:

Family members, including grandparents, siblings, and extended family, also play an essential role in providing emotional support. Their involvement can help create a nurturing and supportive environment for the new mother.

1. **Offering Practical Help**: Family members can provide practical assistance with household tasks, cooking, and childcare. This support allows the mother to focus on her recovery and the baby. It is important for family members to offer help in a way that respects the mother's wishes and boundaries.

2. **Providing Emotional Support**: Like partners, family members can offer a listening ear and emotional support. Sharing positive experiences, offering comfort, and being a source of encouragement can help alleviate feelings of isolation and stress.

3. **Respecting Boundaries**: While family members may want to be involved in the care of the new baby, it is crucial to respect the parents' boundaries and parenting choices. Offering support without imposing opinions or advice helps create a harmonious environment.

4. **Recognizing the Signs of Distress**: Family members should also be aware of the signs of postpartum mental health issues. If they notice concerning behaviors or symptoms, they should approach the situation with compassion and encourage the mother to seek professional help.

Creating a Supportive Environment:

Creating a supportive environment involves open communication, mutual respect, and a willingness to adapt to the changing needs of the new family. This includes:

1. **Open Communication**: Encouraging open and honest communication about feelings, needs, and expectations can prevent misunderstandings and build a stronger support system.

2. **Flexibility and Patience**: The postpartum period is a time of adjustment, and flexibility is key. Partners and family members should be patient with the mother and understand that her needs and emotions may change.

3. **Educating Themselves**: Partners and family members can educate themselves about postpartum mental health to better understand what the mother may be experiencing. This knowledge can help them provide more effective support.

Therapy and Counseling Options

The postpartum period can be a challenging time for many new mothers, with emotional and mental health challenges ranging from the baby blues to more severe conditions like postpartum depression and anxiety. Therapy and counseling offer valuable support and treatment options for those experiencing distress during this time. Various therapeutic approaches can be tailored to meet the specific needs of new mothers, helping them navigate the complexities of postpartum mental health.

Types of Therapy and Counseling:

1. **Cognitive-Behavioral Therapy (CBT)**: CBT is one of the most widely used therapeutic approaches for postpartum mental health issues. It focuses on identifying and changing negative thought patterns and behaviors that contribute to emotional distress. In the context of postpartum depression or anxiety, CBT can help mothers challenge irrational beliefs, such as feeling inadequate or fearing harm to their baby. Techniques such as cognitive restructuring, exposure therapy, and behavioral activation are commonly used. CBT is typically structured, goal-oriented, and time-limited, making it a practical choice for new mothers who may have limited time.

2. **Interpersonal Therapy (IPT)**: IPT is a short-term therapy that focuses on improving interpersonal relationships and communication skills. It is particularly effective for postpartum depression, as it addresses the social and relational factors that can contribute to emotional distress. IPT helps mothers navigate changes in their relationships, such as the transition to parenthood, shifts in partner dynamics, and adjustments in social roles. By improving communication and relationship skills, IPT aims to reduce symptoms of depression and enhance social support.

3. **Psychodynamic Therapy**: Psychodynamic therapy explores unconscious processes and past experiences that influence current behavior and emotions. This therapy is more exploratory and may delve into issues related to early childhood, family dynamics, and unresolved conflicts. For postpartum mothers, psychodynamic therapy can provide insights into how past experiences shape

their current emotional responses and parenting style. This approach can be longer-term and may require a greater time commitment.

4. **Mindfulness-Based Therapies**: Mindfulness-based approaches, such as Mindfulness-Based Cognitive Therapy (MBCT) and Mindfulness-Based Stress Reduction (MBSR), incorporate mindfulness practices to help individuals become more aware of their thoughts, feelings, and bodily sensations. These therapies teach mothers to observe their thoughts without judgment and develop a more compassionate relationship with themselves. Mindfulness practices can be particularly helpful in managing anxiety, stress, and intrusive thoughts.

5. **Support Groups and Group Therapy**: Support groups and group therapy provide a sense of community and shared experience among new mothers facing similar challenges. Group settings offer a supportive environment where mothers can share their experiences, gain insights, and learn coping strategies. Group therapy is typically facilitated by a mental health professional and may focus on specific issues, such as postpartum depression or anxiety, breastfeeding challenges, or parenting stress.

6. **Couples Therapy**: The transition to parenthood can place significant strain on relationships. Couples therapy provides a space for partners to address issues related to communication, intimacy, and shared responsibilities. It can help couples strengthen their relationship, improve conflict resolution skills, and navigate the challenges of parenting together.

Accessing Therapy and Counseling:

New mothers seeking therapy or counseling have several options for accessing services:

1. **In-Person Sessions**: Traditional in-person therapy involves meeting with a therapist at a clinic or office. This option allows for direct, face-to-face interaction and may be preferable for those who benefit from in-person communication.

2. **Teletherapy**: Teletherapy, or online therapy, has become increasingly popular and accessible. It offers the convenience of receiving therapy from home, which can be particularly beneficial for new mothers with limited mobility or childcare responsibilities. Teletherapy can be conducted via video calls, phone calls, or messaging platforms.

3. **Community Resources**: Many communities offer resources for new mothers, including support groups, parenting classes, and mental health services. Community health centers, hospitals, and nonprofit organizations may provide low-cost or sliding-scale options.

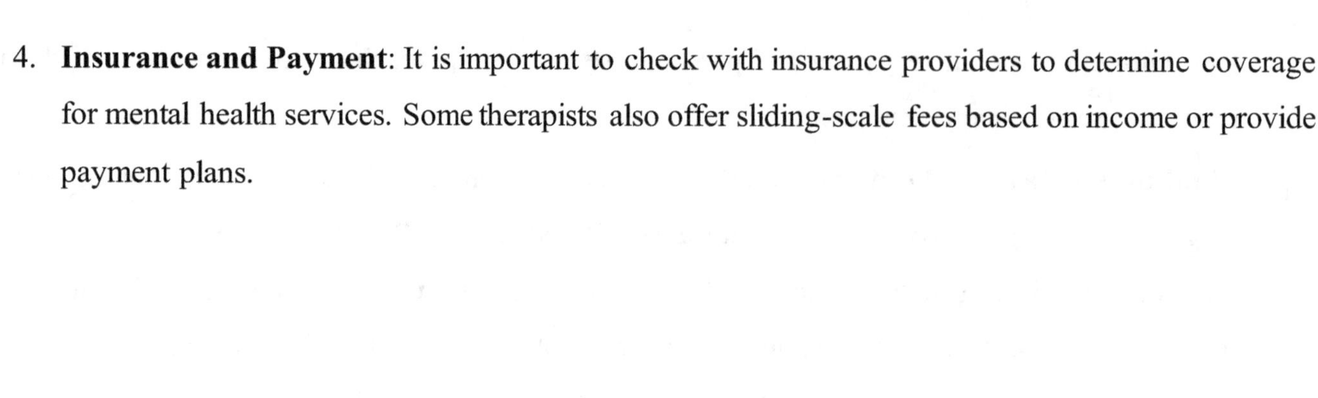

4. **Insurance and Payment**: It is important to check with insurance providers to determine coverage for mental health services. Some therapists also offer sliding-scale fees based on income or provide payment plans.

CHAPTER 4: NUTRITION AND HYDRATION

Nutritional Needs for Recovery

The postpartum period is a time of significant physical and emotional adjustment for new mothers. Proper nutrition during this time is crucial for healing, replenishing nutrient stores, and supporting overall wellbeing. The body undergoes tremendous changes during pregnancy and childbirth, and a balanced diet can help facilitate a smooth recovery.

Caloric Intake and Macronutrients: After giving birth, a woman's body requires additional calories to recover from childbirth and, if breastfeeding, to produce milk. The exact number of extra calories needed can vary based on individual factors such as age, metabolism, and activity level. However, breastfeeding mothers generally need an additional 300-500 calories per day.

Proteins: Protein is essential for tissue repair and muscle recovery, making it a critical component of the postpartum diet. High-quality protein sources include lean meats, poultry, fish, eggs, dairy products, legumes, and nuts. Protein also plays a vital role in the production of enzymes and hormones, which can help regulate mood and energy levels.

Carbohydrates: Carbohydrates provide the primary source of energy for the body. It's important to focus on complex carbohydrates, such as whole grains, fruits, and vegetables, which provide a steady supply of energy and are rich in fiber, vitamins, and minerals. Fiber is particularly beneficial for preventing constipation, a common issue during the postpartum period.

Fats: Healthy fats are necessary for hormone production, brain health, and overall cellular function. Incorporating sources of unsaturated fats, such as avocados, nuts, seeds, and olive oil, can support these bodily functions. Omega-3 fatty acids, found in fatty fish like salmon and mackerel, are especially important for reducing inflammation and supporting brain health.

Micronutrients: Alongside macronutrients, micronutrients like vitamins and minerals are vital for recovery. Iron is particularly important to replenish blood lost during childbirth and prevent anemia. Good sources of iron include red meat, poultry, fish, lentils, beans, and fortified cereals. Consuming vitamin C rich foods, such as citrus fruits, alongside iron-rich foods can enhance absorption.

Calcium is another crucial nutrient, especially for breastfeeding mothers, as it supports bone health. Dairy products, leafy green vegetables, and fortified plant-based milks are excellent sources of calcium. Vitamin D, necessary for calcium absorption, can be obtained through sun exposure and foods like fatty fish, fortified dairy products, and egg yolks.

Hydration: Staying well-hydrated is essential for overall health and recovery. Adequate hydration is particularly important for breastfeeding mothers, as it supports milk production. Water should be the primary source of hydration, but herbal teas and broths can also contribute to fluid intake.

Meal Planning and Convenience: The demands of caring for a newborn can make it challenging to prioritize nutritious meals. Planning and preparing meals in advance can help ensure that nutritious foods are readily available. Simple, nutrient-dense meals and snacks, such as yogurt with fruit, whole-grain toast with avocado, or a smoothie with leafy greens, can provide the necessary nutrients without requiring extensive preparation.

Special Dietary Considerations (e.g., Anemia, C-section Recovery)

The postpartum period often involves specific dietary considerations, especially for women who have experienced certain conditions or delivery methods, such as anemia or a cesarean section (C-section). Tailoring nutrition to address these specific needs can significantly enhance recovery and overall wellbeing.

Anemia: Anemia is a common concern postpartum, particularly for women who experienced significant blood loss during childbirth. Iron deficiency anemia, characterized by low levels of hemoglobin in the blood, can lead to symptoms such as fatigue, weakness, and dizziness. Addressing this condition through diet is crucial.

Iron Intake: To combat anemia, increasing dietary iron intake is essential. There are two types of dietary iron: heme iron, found in animal products, and non-heme iron, found in plant-based foods. Heme iron is more readily absorbed by the body. Good sources of heme iron include red meat, poultry, and fish. Nonheme iron sources include lentils, beans, tofu, spinach, and fortified cereals. Enhancing non-heme iron absorption can be achieved by consuming vitamin C-rich foods, such as citrus fruits, berries, bell peppers, and tomatoes, alongside iron-rich meals.

Folate and Vitamin B12: These nutrients are also important for addressing anemia. Folate, or vitamin B9, is crucial for the production of healthy red blood cells and can be found in leafy greens, legumes, nuts, and fortified grains. Vitamin B12, essential for red blood cell formation and neurological function, is found in animal products such as meat, dairy, and eggs. For vegetarians or vegans, fortified foods or supplements may be necessary to ensure adequate intake.

C-Section Recovery: Recovery from a C-section requires additional nutritional support due to the surgical nature of the delivery. Proper nutrition can aid in wound healing, reduce inflammation, and prevent infections.

Protein for Tissue Repair: Adequate protein intake is critical for wound healing and tissue repair. Good protein sources include lean meats, fish, eggs, dairy products, legumes, and nuts. Consuming a variety of protein sources ensures a supply of all essential amino acids needed for recovery.

Vitamin C and Collagen: Vitamin C is vital for collagen synthesis, a key protein in wound healing. Consuming foods rich in vitamin C, such as citrus fruits, strawberries, bell peppers, and broccoli, can support this process.

Zinc for Immune Function: Zinc plays a significant role in immune function and wound healing. It is found in meats, shellfish, dairy products, legumes, and seeds. Ensuring adequate zinc intake can help prevent infections and promote quicker healing.

Anti-inflammatory Foods: Including anti-inflammatory foods in the diet can help manage post-surgical inflammation. Omega-3 fatty acids, found in fatty fish-like salmon and mackerel, flaxseeds, chia seeds, and walnuts, are known for their anti-inflammatory properties. Incorporating these foods can aid in reducing inflammation and supporting recovery.

Hydration and Fiber: Hydration is crucial for overall recovery, and maintaining bowel regularity is important, particularly after a C-section when abdominal muscles may be tender. High-fiber foods, such as whole grains, fruits, vegetables, and legumes, along with adequate fluid intake, can help prevent constipation.

The Importance of Hydration

Hydration is a fundamental component of postpartum recovery, playing a crucial role in overall health, physical recovery, and the well-being of new mothers. Adequate fluid intake is essential for various physiological processes, including regulating body temperature, maintaining blood volume, supporting metabolic functions, and aiding in digestion. During the postpartum period, the importance of hydration becomes even more pronounced, particularly for breastfeeding mothers.

Physical Recovery: After childbirth, the body needs to repair tissues, heal from any birth-related injuries, and return to its pre-pregnancy state. Water is a critical component of this healing process, as it helps maintain adequate blood volume, which is essential for delivering nutrients to tissues and removing waste products. Proper hydration also aids in the function of organs and systems that may have been stressed during pregnancy and delivery.

Breastfeeding and Milk Production: For breastfeeding mothers, hydration is directly linked to milk production. Breast milk is composed of about 87% water, making it essential for breastfeeding mothers to consume enough fluids to produce sufficient milk for their infants. Dehydration can lead to a decrease in milk supply, which can affect the baby's nutrition and growth. Thus, breastfeeding mothers need to increase their fluid intake to meet the demands of milk production.

Managing Postpartum Edema: Many women experience postpartum edema, a condition characterized by swelling due to fluid retention. This swelling is often seen in the extremities, such as the hands, feet, and legs. While it might seem counterintuitive, drinking plenty of water can help reduce this swelling. Adequate hydration helps the body flush out excess sodium and fluids, which can alleviate swelling and discomfort.

Hormonal Balance: The postpartum period is marked by significant hormonal changes that can affect fluid balance in the body. For example, the hormone oxytocin, which is released during breastfeeding and helps with uterine contractions, can also influence water retention. Staying well-hydrated helps the body manage these hormonal shifts and maintain a stable internal environment.

Mental and Emotional Health: Dehydration can negatively impact mental and emotional health, contributing to symptoms such as fatigue, irritability, and difficulty concentrating. The demands of caring for a newborn can be emotionally and physically exhausting, and dehydration can exacerbate these challenges. Proper hydration supports cognitive function, mood stability, and overall mental clarity, helping new mothers cope better with the stresses of postpartum life.

How to Stay Hydrated:

1. **Water**: Water is the best choice for hydration. New mothers should aim to drink at least 8-10 glasses of water per day, with adjustments based on individual needs and circumstances, such as breastfeeding or increased physical activity.

2. **Other Fluids**: While water should be the primary source of hydration, other fluids such as herbal teas, milk, and natural fruit juices can also contribute to daily fluid intake. However, it's important to limit caffeine and sugary drinks, as they can have diuretic effects and may not be as hydrating.

3. **Monitoring Hydration**: Keeping track of fluid intake can help ensure adequate hydration. Simple methods include using a water bottle with measurement markings, setting reminders to drink water, and paying attention to signs of dehydration, such as dark-colored urine, dry mouth, or dizziness.

4. **Incorporating Hydrating Foods**: Certain foods have high water content and can contribute to overall hydration. Examples include fruits like watermelon, strawberries, and oranges, as well as vegetables like cucumbers, celery, and bell peppers.

Supplements and Vitamins

During the postpartum period, nutritional supplements and vitamins can play a significant role in supporting recovery, addressing specific deficiencies, and promoting overall health. While a well-balanced diet should be the primary source of nutrients, supplements can provide additional support, especially if dietary intake is insufficient or if specific health conditions arise.

Postpartum Multivitamins: Postpartum multivitamins are designed to meet the increased nutritional needs of new mothers. These supplements often contain a combination of essential vitamins and minerals that support overall health and recovery. Key components of postpartum multivitamins may include:

1. **Vitamin D**: Supports calcium absorption and bone health. Many women require additional vitamin D, especially if they have limited sun exposure.

2. **Iron**: Essential for replenishing iron stores depleted during childbirth. Iron supplements can help prevent or address postpartum anemia.

3. **Calcium**: Important for maintaining bone strength, especially for breastfeeding mothers who transfer calcium to their infants through breast milk.

4. **B Vitamins**: Includes folate (vitamin B9), vitamin B12, and other B vitamins that support energy production, red blood cell formation, and overall vitality.

5. **Omega-3 Fatty Acids**: Often included for their anti-inflammatory properties and benefits for mood stabilization. Omega-3s can also support brain health and cognitive function.

Specific Supplements:

1. **Iron Supplements**: Iron is critical for replenishing blood stores and preventing anemia. Postpartum women, particularly those who experienced significant blood loss during delivery, may benefit from iron supplements. It is essential to take iron supplements as directed by a healthcare provider, as excessive iron can cause gastrointestinal issues.

2. **Calcium and Vitamin D**: These supplements are important for bone health, particularly if dietary intake is insufficient. Vitamin D enhances calcium absorption, and a combination of calcium and vitamin D can support bone strength and overall health.

3. **Probiotics**: Probiotics can support gut health and immune function. After childbirth and antibiotic use (if applicable), probiotics may help restore a healthy balance of gut bacteria. Probiotic supplements can aid digestion and improve overall gut health.

4. **Fish Oil**: Rich in omega-3 fatty acids, fish oil supplements can support mental health, reduce inflammation, and promote heart health. Omega-3s are also beneficial for breastfeeding mothers, as they support the development of the baby's brain and eyes.

5. **Herbal Supplements**: Some herbal supplements, such as fenugreek and blessed thistle, are used to support milk production in breastfeeding mothers. However, it is crucial to consult with a healthcare provider before using herbal supplements, as they can interact with medications or have side effects.

Considerations and Recommendations:

1. **Consult a Healthcare Provider**: Before starting any new supplements, it is essential to consult with a healthcare provider. They can assess individual needs, recommend appropriate supplements, and ensure there are no contraindications with existing medications or health conditions.

2. **Quality and Safety**: Choose high-quality supplements from reputable brands to ensure safety and effectiveness. Look for products that have been tested for purity and potency.

3. **Balanced Diet First**: While supplements can be beneficial, they should not replace a balanced diet. A varied and nutrient-dense diet remains the foundation of postpartum nutrition.

Eating for Breastfeeding

Breastfeeding is a vital aspect of postpartum recovery and infant care, and proper nutrition is crucial for supporting both the mother's health and the baby's growth and development. The nutritional needs of breastfeeding mothers are unique, and eating a well-balanced diet can help ensure an adequate milk supply while promoting overall well-being.

Increased Caloric Needs: Breastfeeding mothers require additional calories to support milk production. On average, breastfeeding can increase daily caloric needs by approximately 300-500 calories. These extra calories should come from nutrient-dense foods that provide essential vitamins and minerals, rather than empty calories.

Macronutrients:

1. **Proteins**: Protein is essential for milk production and overall health. High-quality protein sources, such as lean meats, poultry, fish, eggs, dairy products, legumes, and nuts, should be included in the diet. Protein helps repair tissues, support immune function, and maintain energy levels.

2. **Carbohydrates**: Carbohydrates provide the energy needed for milk production and daily activities. Focus on complex carbohydrates, such as whole grains, fruits, and vegetables, which

provide sustained energy and essential nutrients. Fiber-rich foods can also help prevent constipation, which can be a common issue postpartum.

3. **Fats**: Healthy fats are important for brain health, hormone regulation, and overall energy. Sources of healthy fats include avocados, nuts, seeds, olive oil, and fatty fish. Omega-3 fatty acids, in particular, are beneficial for both the mother and baby, supporting brain development and reducing inflammation.

Micronutrients:

1. **Calcium**: Calcium is crucial for bone health, especially for breastfeeding mothers who transfer calcium to their infants through breast milk. Dairy products, fortified plant-based milks, leafy green vegetables, and almonds are good sources of calcium.

2. **Iron**: Iron is important for maintaining energy levels and preventing anemia. Include iron-rich foods such as lean meats, poultry, fish, beans, lentils, and fortified cereals. Consuming vitamin C rich foods alongside iron sources can enhance absorption.

3. **Vitamin D**: Vitamin D supports calcium absorption and immune function. Breastfeeding mothers may need to ensure adequate vitamin D intake through sunlight exposure, fortified foods, or supplements if necessary.

4. **Vitamin A**: Vitamin A is important for vision, immune function, and skin health. Sources include orange and yellow vegetables (carrots, sweet potatoes), leafy greens, and dairy products.

Hydration: Staying well-hydrated is essential for milk production and overall health. Drinking plenty of water throughout the day is crucial, as dehydration can reduce milk supply and affect energy levels. Herbal teas and soups can also contribute to hydration, but it is important to limit caffeine and sugary beverages.

Balanced Meals and Snacks: Eating regular, balanced meals and snacks can help maintain energy levels and support milk production. Plan meals that include a variety of food groups, such as lean proteins, whole grains, fruits, and vegetables. Healthy snacks, like yogurt, fruit, nuts, and whole-grain crackers, can provide additional nutrients and keep hunger at bay.

Avoiding Certain Foods: While a varied diet is important, some foods and substances should be limited or avoided during breastfeeding. These include:

1. **Caffeine**: Excessive caffeine intake can affect the baby's sleep patterns and may be associated with irritability. It is generally recommended to limit caffeine consumption to 300-500 mg per day (about 2-3 cups of coffee).

2. **Alcohol**: Alcohol can pass into breast milk and affect the baby. It is advisable to limit alcohol consumption and wait at least 2-3 hours after drinking before breastfeeding.

3. **Potential Allergens**: Some foods, such as peanuts or shellfish, may cause allergic reactions in sensitive infants. If there are concerns about allergies, consult with a healthcare provider for guidance.

CHAPTER 5: BREASTFEEDING AND LACTATION

Getting Started with Breastfeeding

Breastfeeding is a natural and beneficial way to nourish a newborn, but it can require some learning and practice for both mother and baby. The initial steps in breastfeeding are crucial for establishing a successful feeding routine and ensuring a positive experience for both. Here's a comprehensive guide to getting started with breastfeeding.

The First Latch: The first few hours after birth are an ideal time to initiate breastfeeding. This period is often referred to as the "golden hour," where the newborn is alert and more likely to latch onto the breast. Skin-to-skin contact during this time helps to regulate the baby's body temperature, heart rate, and breathing, and also encourages the baby to seek out the breast. It's essential to find a comfortable position, whether it's the cradle hold, cross-cradle hold, or football hold, to support the baby and allow for a good latch.

Positioning and Latch: A proper latch is key to successful breastfeeding. To achieve a good latch, the baby's mouth should cover not just the nipple but a significant portion of the areola, ensuring that the baby's lips are flanged outwards and the tongue is under the breast. This allows the baby to compress the milk ducts effectively and minimize nipple discomfort for the mother. A shallow latch can lead to sore nipples and inefficient milk transfer. Signs of a good latch include rhythmic sucking, swallowing sounds, and a lack of pain for the mother.

Feeding Cues and Frequency: Newborns often feed frequently, approximately 8-12 times in a 24-hour period. It's important to recognize feeding cues, which include rooting (turning the head towards something that touches their cheek), sucking on hands, and making sucking noises. Crying is typically a late sign of hunger. Frequent feeding helps stimulate milk production and ensures the baby receives adequate nutrition.

Milk Production and Let-Down: Initially, the breasts produce colostrum, a thick, nutrient-rich fluid that is perfect for the newborn's small stomach and provides essential antibodies. Within a few days, the milk will "come in," becoming more abundant and transitioning to mature milk. The let-down reflex is a key component of breastfeeding, where the release of oxytocin causes the milk to flow from the alveoli (milkproducing glands) through the ducts to the nipple. Mothers may feel a tingling sensation during let-down, though it can vary widely in intensity.

Support and Education: Breastfeeding can come with a learning curve, and seeking support can make a significant difference. Lactation consultants, who are trained professionals in breastfeeding support, can offer personalized guidance and help address any issues with latching, positioning, and milk supply. Many hospitals and clinics offer lactation services, and there are also numerous online resources and support groups for breastfeeding mothers.

Challenges and Persistence: It's important to acknowledge that breastfeeding may not always be straightforward. Issues such as sore nipples, engorgement, or difficulty latching can arise. It's crucial to address these challenges early with the help of healthcare providers or lactation consultants. Persistence and patience are key, as breastfeeding often becomes easier with practice and support.

Overcoming Common Challenges

Breastfeeding, while natural, can present a range of challenges for new mothers. These challenges can sometimes feel overwhelming, but understanding common issues and knowing how to address them can lead to a more successful and enjoyable breastfeeding journey. Here's a look at some of the most common challenges and practical solutions.

Sore Nipples: Sore or cracked nipples are a frequent issue for new breastfeeding mothers. They often result from an improper latch, where the baby's mouth is not positioned correctly on the breast. To alleviate this, it's crucial to ensure that the baby latches deeply, covering more of the areola than just the nipple. Using lanolin-based creams or expressed breast milk can also help soothe sore nipples. If soreness persists, consulting a lactation consultant can provide specific advice on adjusting the latch and positioning.

Engorgement: Breast engorgement occurs when the breasts become overly full, hard, and painful. This can happen when milk first comes in or if the baby is not feeding frequently enough. To manage engorgement, it's important to feed the baby often or express milk to relieve fullness. Warm compresses and gentle massage before feeding can help stimulate milk flow, while cold compresses after feeding can reduce swelling. Wearing a well-fitting, supportive bra can also provide comfort.

Low Milk Supply: Concerns about low milk supply are common among breastfeeding mothers. However, true low milk supply is relatively rare. Often, the perception of insufficient milk arises from misunderstanding normal feeding patterns or growth spurts. To boost milk supply, mothers should nurse frequently, as milk production works on a supply-and-demand basis. Ensuring the baby has a good latch, staying hydrated, and maintaining a balanced diet are also crucial. In some cases, herbal supplements like fenugreek or medications may be recommended by a healthcare provider.

Oversupply and Fast Let-Down: An oversupply of milk can lead to issues such as forceful let-down, where milk flows too quickly for the baby to manage. This can cause the baby to cough or choke during feeding and lead to symptoms like gas or fussiness. To manage oversupply, mothers can try feeding from one breast per feeding session to regulate milk production. Allowing the baby to nurse at a comfortable pace and using positions like a laid-back position can also help control the flow of milk.

Mastitis: Mastitis is an inflammation of the breast tissue, often caused by an infection. Symptoms include breast pain, redness, swelling, fever, and flu-like symptoms. It is crucial to continue breastfeeding during mastitis, as milk removal helps clear the infection. Applying warm compresses, gentle breast massage, and ensuring frequent, effective milk removal can aid in recovery. If symptoms persist or worsen, medical treatment, including antibiotics, may be necessary.

Blocked Ducts: Blocked milk ducts can occur when milk is not fully drained from the breast, leading to a painful lump. To relieve a blocked duct, mothers should continue breastfeeding, as frequent milk removal can help. Warm compresses and massage toward the nipple during feeding can assist in clearing the blockage. Changing feeding positions can also ensure all ducts are emptied effectively.

Breastfeeding in Public: Some mothers may feel uncomfortable breastfeeding in public due to concerns about privacy or societal attitudes. Planning ahead by wearing breastfeeding-friendly clothing and using nursing covers can provide discretion. It's also helpful to practice breastfeeding at home to build confidence. Remember, breastfeeding is a natural and legally protected right in many places.

Emotional and Mental Health: The emotional aspects of breastfeeding can also present challenges. Feelings of frustration, guilt, or anxiety are common, especially if breastfeeding does not go as planned. It's important for mothers to seek support from healthcare providers, lactation consultants, family, and friends. Joining breastfeeding support groups can provide encouragement and practical advice from others experiencing similar challenges.

Benefits of Breastfeeding for Mother and Baby

Breastfeeding offers a multitude of benefits for both the mother and the baby, encompassing nutritional, immunological, psychological, and economic aspects. These benefits are well-documented and widely recognized by healthcare professionals and organizations, making breastfeeding the recommended method of infant feeding whenever possible. Here's an in-depth look at the numerous advantages of breastfeeding.

Nutritional Benefits for the Baby: Breast milk is the optimal source of nutrition for infants. It is uniquely composed to meet the nutritional needs of a baby, containing the perfect balance of proteins, fats, vitamins, and minerals. Moreover, the composition of breast milk changes over time to match the growing needs of the infant, providing the right nutrients at every stage of development.

Immunological Protection: One of the most significant benefits of breastfeeding is the immune protection it offers to the baby. Breast milk contains antibodies, particularly immunoglobulin A (IgA), that help protect the infant from infections by forming a protective layer on the mucous membranes in the baby's intestines, nose, and throat. This protection helps reduce the incidence of illnesses such as respiratory infections, ear infections, gastrointestinal infections, and urinary tract infections. Additionally, breastfeeding has been associated with a lower risk of sudden infant death syndrome (SIDS).

Bonding and Emotional Benefits: Breastfeeding fosters a unique bond between mother and baby. The close physical contact, skin-to-skin touch, and eye contact during breastfeeding promote emotional connection and attachment. This bonding is not only comforting for the baby but also enhances the mother's emotional well-being, contributing to a stronger mother-infant relationship.

Health Benefits for the mother: Breastfeeding offers significant health benefits for mothers. It helps the uterus contract and return to its pre-pregnancy size, reducing postpartum bleeding. Breastfeeding also burns extra calories, which can aid in postpartum weight loss. Long-term benefits include a reduced risk of breast and ovarian cancers, type 2 diabetes, and cardiovascular disease. The release of oxytocin during breastfeeding promotes a sense of relaxation and well-being, which can help reduce stress and lower the risk of postpartum depression.

Cognitive and Developmental Advantages: Breastfeeding has been linked to improved cognitive development in children. Studies suggest that breastfed children may have higher IQ scores and better academic performance later in life compared to their formula-fed peers. The long-chain polyunsaturated fatty acids found in breast milk, particularly DHA (docosahexaenoic acid), are crucial for brain development and visual acuity.

Convenience and Economic Benefits: Breastfeeding is convenient and cost-effective. It requires no preparation, is always at the right temperature, and is readily available wherever the mother and baby are. This convenience is particularly valuable during night feedings or when traveling. Economically, breastfeeding can save families significant money compared to the cost of formula feeding. It also reduces healthcare costs by decreasing the likelihood of illnesses in both mother and baby, leading to fewer doctor visits and hospitalizations.

Environmental Impact: Breastfeeding is environmentally friendly, producing no waste from packaging or manufacturing processes, and reducing the carbon footprint associated with the production, transportation, and disposal of formula products.

Pumping and Storing Breast Milk

Pumping and storing breast milk is a practical solution for many breastfeeding mothers, providing flexibility and ensuring that babies receive the benefits of breast milk even when direct breastfeeding is not possible. Whether returning to work, dealing with latching issues, or needing to maintain milk supply, understanding the process of pumping and storing breast milk is essential.

Choosing a Breast Pump: Selecting the right breast pump depends on individual needs. There are three main types of breast pumps: manual, electric, and hospital-grade. Manual pumps are operated by hand and are portable, making them suitable for occasional use. Electric pumps, available in single or double models, are powered by electricity or batteries and are ideal for regular use. Hospital-grade pumps are the most efficient and are often used in medical settings or for mothers with low milk supply or preterm infants. They are available for rental through hospitals and lactation consultants.

Pumping Techniques: To maximize milk expression, it's important to pump in a comfortable, relaxed environment. Mothers should start by massaging the breasts to stimulate milk flow. Using a warm compress before pumping can also help. When using an electric pump, it's recommended to start at a low suction level and gradually increase to a comfortable setting. Pumping sessions should last about 15-20 minutes per breast or until the milk flow slows down. Double pumping can save time and may increase milk production.

Storing Breast Milk: Proper storage of expressed breast milk is crucial for maintaining its quality and safety. Breast milk can be stored in clean, BPA-free bottles or breast milk storage bags. It's important to label containers with the date and time of expression. Freshly pumped milk can be stored at room temperature (up to 77°F or 25°C) for up to four hours, in the refrigerator (at 39°F or 4°C) for up to four days, and in the freezer (at 0°F or -18°C) for up to six months. For deep freezer storage (at -4°F or -20°C), milk can be kept for 12 months, although usage within six months is recommended for optimal quality.

Thawing and Warming Breast Milk: Thaw frozen milk in the refrigerator overnight or by placing the container in a bowl of warm water. It's important to avoid using a microwave, as it can create hot spots and destroy beneficial nutrients. Gently swirl the milk to mix any separated layers. Breast milk can be warmed by placing the bottle in warm water or using a bottle warmer. Before feeding, test the temperature on the inside of your wrist to ensure it's not too hot.

Cleaning and Maintenance: Proper cleaning of pump parts and storage containers is essential to prevent contamination. After each use, all parts that come into contact with breast milk should be washed with warm, soapy water and thoroughly rinsed. Many pump parts are dishwasher safe, but always check the manufacturer's instructions. Sterilizing pump parts is recommended periodically, especially for newborns or preterm infants. This can be done by boiling, using a microwave steam sterilizer, or employing a sterilizing solution.

Maintaining Milk Supply: Regular pumping is crucial to maintaining milk supply, especially if direct breastfeeding is reduced or stopped. It's recommended to pump at the same frequency as the baby's feeding schedule. Nighttime pumping can be particularly beneficial, as prolactin levels, which promote milk production, are higher at night. Staying hydrated, eating a balanced diet, and getting enough rest are also important for sustaining milk supply.

Pumping at Work: For working mothers, planning and organization are key to successful pumping. It's important to know your rights, as many workplaces are required to provide a private space and reasonable break times for pumping. Investing in a good-quality, portable pump and a cooler bag for milk storage can make pumping at work more manageable.

Conclusion: Pumping and storing breast milk offers breastfeeding mothers flexibility and the ability to continue providing breast milk when direct breastfeeding is not possible. By understanding the techniques for efficient pumping, proper storage guidelines, and maintenance of equipment, mothers can ensure their babies receive the best possible nutrition. Whether pumping occasionally or exclusively, the benefits of providing breast milk are invaluable for both mother and baby.

Weaning and Transitioning

Weaning, the process of transitioning a baby from breast milk to other forms of nutrition, is a significant milestone in a child's development. This transition can be emotional and complex, as it involves physical, psychological, and logistical considerations. Whether the weaning process is initiated by the mother or the baby, it is important to approach it with sensitivity and awareness of the child's needs.

Timing of Weaning: The timing of weaning varies widely depending on cultural, personal, and health factors. The World Health Organization (WHO) recommends exclusive breastfeeding for the first six months of life, followed by continued breastfeeding along with appropriate complementary foods for up to two years or beyond. However, the decision to wean is highly individual and can occur anytime based on the mother's or child's readiness. Some children naturally lose interest in breastfeeding as they begin to consume more solid foods, while others may breastfeed well into the toddler years.

Gradual Weaning: Gradual weaning is generally the most comfortable approach for both mother and child. It involves slowly reducing breastfeeding sessions, which helps the mother's body gradually decrease milk production and reduces the risk of engorgement and mastitis. This method also allows the child time to adjust emotionally and nutritionally to new sources of nourishment. For example, one feeding session can be replaced with a bottle of pumped milk, formula, or a nutritious snack, depending on the child's age.

Substitute Nutrition: As breastfeeding decreases, it's essential to ensure the child receives adequate nutrition from other sources. For infants under one year, breast milk or formula should remain the primary source of nutrition. After one year, whole cow's milk can be introduced along with a varied diet of solid foods, including fruits, vegetables, grains, proteins, and healthy fats. It's important to offer a balanced diet that meets the child's nutritional needs, including sufficient iron, calcium, and other essential nutrients.

Comfort and Emotional Support: Weaning can be an emotional process for both mother and child. The child may seek comfort from breastfeeding, and its cessation can be distressing. To ease the transition, mothers can offer extra cuddles, attention, and comfort in other ways. Maintaining a nurturing bedtime routine, offering a favorite blanket or toy, and spending quality time together can help the child feel secure. Mothers should also be mindful of their own emotions, as weaning can bring feelings of sadness or loss. It's important to acknowledge these feelings and seek support from friends, family, or support groups if needed.

Handling Challenges: Weaning can sometimes bring challenges, such as resistance from the child, discomfort from engorged breasts, or concerns about adequate nutrition. If a child is resistant to weaning, it may be helpful to change the daily routine, offering distractions or new activities during typical breastfeeding times. For mothers experiencing engorgement, gradually reducing feedings and expressing milk just enough to relieve discomfort can help. In cases where the child's nutrition is a concern, consulting a pediatrician or nutritionist can provide guidance on appropriate dietary adjustments.

Complete Weaning and Aftercare: Complete weaning occurs when breastfeeding has entirely stopped. This transition may happen gradually or more suddenly, depending on circumstances. After complete weaning, mothers may experience changes in their breasts, including a reduction in size and potential changes in texture. It's important to continue regular breast self-examinations and consult a healthcare provider if any concerns arise.

Special Considerations: In some cases, weaning may need to be approached differently, such as when a mother or child has health issues, or in cases of premature weaning due to medical reasons. In these situations, it's important to work closely with healthcare professionals to ensure the well-being of both mother and child.

CHAPTER 6: PHYSICAL FITNESS AND EXERCISE

When to Start Exercising

The postpartum period is a time of recovery and adjustment for new mothers, and understanding when to start exercising is crucial for a safe return to physical activity. While it's beneficial to reintroduce exercise for physical and mental well-being, the timing should be personalized, taking into account the type of delivery, any complications, and overall recovery.

General Guidelines: Typically, healthcare providers recommend waiting until the six-week postpartum check-up before starting any formal exercise program. This allows time for the body to heal, particularly if there were complications such as a cesarean section, perineal tearing, or postpartum hemorrhage. However, the exact timing can vary depending on individual circumstances. For women who experienced a normal vaginal delivery without complications, gentle activities like walking can usually be resumed sooner, often as early as a few days postpartum, provided they feel ready.

Signs of Readiness: Physical readiness for exercise postpartum depends on several factors, including the absence of pain, bleeding, or discomfort. Key signs indicating readiness include the cessation of postpartum bleeding (lochia), the healing of any perineal stitches, and the general feeling of physical readiness. Emotional readiness is also important; new mothers should feel mentally prepared and have the energy to incorporate exercise into their daily routine.

Consulting with Healthcare Providers: It's essential to consult with a healthcare provider before starting any exercise regimen postpartum. This is particularly crucial for mothers who experienced complications during childbirth or pregnancy, such as preeclampsia, gestational diabetes, or severe tearing. Healthcare providers can offer personalized advice and ensure that any exercise program is safe and appropriate.

Initial Focus: The initial focus should be on gentle, low-impact activities that promote overall well-being without putting too much strain on the body. Walking is an excellent starting point, as it helps improve cardiovascular health, enhances mood, and can be done with the baby in a stroller, making it convenient.

Light stretching and breathing exercises can also aid in relaxation and stress relief.

Listening to the Body: New mothers should pay close attention to their bodies and avoid pushing themselves too hard, too soon. Signs of overexertion can include increased bleeding, pain, or discomfort, particularly in the abdominal or pelvic region. It's important to gradually increase the intensity and duration of exercise based on how the body responds, rather than adhering to a fixed schedule.

The Role of Core and Pelvic Floor Recovery: Special attention should be given to core and pelvic floor recovery, as these areas undergo significant changes during pregnancy and childbirth. Weakness in the abdominal and pelvic floor muscles can lead to issues such as back pain, urinary incontinence, and pelvic organ prolapse. Initial exercises should include gentle pelvic floor exercises (Kegels) and deep core activation exercises to re-establish strength and function in these critical areas.

Emotional Considerations: The postpartum period can be an emotionally challenging time, and exercise can play a beneficial role in improving mood and reducing stress. However, it's important to approach exercise as a positive and enjoyable activity, rather than as a means to lose weight or regain a prepregnancy body. Focusing on the physical and mental health benefits, rather than appearance, can promote a healthier and more sustainable approach to postpartum fitness.

Safe Postpartum Exercises

Postpartum exercise plays a crucial role in helping new mothers recover from childbirth and regain strength and fitness. However, it is essential to choose safe and appropriate exercises that take into account the unique changes and challenges the body undergoes during the postpartum period. Here's a guide to safe postpartum exercises that can help new mothers rebuild strength, improve mood, and enhance overall well-being.

Walking: Walking is one of the safest and most accessible forms of exercise postpartum. It's a low-impact activity that can be started soon after childbirth, even within the first few days, depending on the mother's comfort level. Walking helps improve cardiovascular health, boosts energy levels, and provides a gentle way to ease back into physical activity. New mothers can start with short walks and gradually increase the duration and intensity as they feel stronger.

Pelvic Floor Exercises (Kegels): The pelvic floor muscles can be weakened by pregnancy and childbirth, leading to issues such as urinary incontinence. Kegel exercises are essential for strengthening these muscles and can be started as soon as comfortable postpartum. To perform Kegels, the mother should contract the pelvic floor muscles as if trying to stop the flow of urine, hold for a few seconds, and then release. Repeating this exercise multiple times a day can help restore strength and function in the pelvic floor.

Deep Breathing and Core Activation: Pregnancy and childbirth can weaken the core muscles, including the deep abdominal muscles. Deep breathing exercises that focus on core activation can help re-engage these muscles. One effective exercise is the "belly breathing" technique, where the mother inhales deeply, allowing the abdomen to expand, then exhales while drawing the belly button toward the spine. This exercise helps activate the transverse abdominis, a key muscle for core stability.

Modified Yoga and Stretching: Gentle yoga and stretching exercises can help improve flexibility, reduce stress, and promote relaxation. However, postpartum mothers should avoid poses that put excessive pressure on the abdomen or involve deep twists and backbends, especially if they have diastasis recti (separation of the abdominal muscles). Poses such as child's pose, cat-cow, and gentle spinal twists can be beneficial for stretching and relaxing the body.

Leg and Glute Exercises: Strengthening the lower body can help new mothers regain stability and balance. Safe exercises include modified squats, lunges, and glute bridges. These exercises help strengthen the legs and glutes without placing excessive strain on the abdominal muscles. It's important to focus on proper form and start with body weight before progressing to using light weights.

Upper Body Strengthening: As mothers often need to lift and carry their babies, building upper body strength is essential. Safe exercises include wall push-ups, modified push-ups, and light weightlifting exercises like bicep curls and shoulder presses. Using resistance bands can also be a gentle way to start strengthening the upper body. It's important to avoid heavy lifting or strenuous upper body exercises until the body is fully healed and strength is gradually rebuilt.

Low-Impact Cardiovascular Exercise: As energy levels and fitness improve, mothers can incorporate low-impact cardiovascular exercises such as stationary cycling, swimming, or using an elliptical machine. These exercises help improve cardiovascular fitness without putting excessive stress on the joints or the recovering pelvic floor.

Rest and Recovery: Rest is an essential component of any postpartum exercise routine. New mothers should listen to their bodies and avoid pushing themselves too hard, especially in the early postpartum weeks. Adequate sleep and nutrition are also critical for recovery and energy levels.

Rebuilding Core and Abdominal Muscles

Rebuilding core and abdominal muscles postpartum is a critical aspect of recovery and regaining strength. The core, which includes the abdominal muscles, back muscles, and pelvic floor, plays a vital role in stability, balance, and overall function. Pregnancy and childbirth can significantly impact these muscles, leading to issues such as diastasis recti, weakened pelvic floor, and back pain. Here's a comprehensive guide to safely and effectively rebuilding core and abdominal strength postpartum.

Understanding Diastasis Recti: Diastasis recti is a common condition where the right and left halves of the abdominal muscles separate during pregnancy, creating a gap. This separation can weaken the core and contribute to a protruding belly. Before starting any core exercises, it's important to check for diastasis recti. This can be done by lying on the back with knees bent, lifting the head slightly, and feeling for a gap along the midline of the abdomen. If a gap is present, exercises should focus on healing the separation rather than traditional ab workouts like crunches, which can exacerbate the condition.

Deep Core Activation: Rebuilding the core starts with activating the deep core muscles, particularly the transverse abdominis (TVA). The TVA acts like a corset, stabilizing the spine and supporting the internal organs. One effective exercise for activating the TVA is the "drawing-in" maneuver. This involves lying on the back with knees bent, inhaling deeply, and then exhaling while pulling the belly button towards the spine, engaging the deep core muscles. This exercise can be performed throughout the day and incorporated into other movements.

Pelvic Tilts: Pelvic tilts are a gentle exercise that helps strengthen the lower back and abdominal muscles. To perform a pelvic tilt, lie on your back with knees bent and feet flat on the floor. Inhale and then exhale while tilting the pelvis upward, flattening the lower back against the floor. Hold for a few seconds, then release. This exercise can help improve core strength and pelvic alignment.

Modified Plank: The plank is an excellent exercise for core strengthening, but it should be modified in the postpartum period to avoid excessive pressure on the abdomen. A modified plank can be performed on the knees instead of the toes, or by leaning against a stable surface like a wall or countertop. Focus on maintaining a straight line from head to hips and engaging the core without letting the lower back sag. Hold the position for a few seconds, gradually increasing the duration as strength improves.

Heel Slides: Heel slides are another gentle exercise for engaging the lower abdominal muscles. Lie on your back with knees bent and feet flat on the floor. Slowly slide one heel away from the body, keeping the core engaged and the lower back flat against the floor. Return to the starting position and repeat with the other leg. This exercise helps strengthen the lower abs and improve coordination.

Leg Raises with Knee Bent: For a more advanced exercise, leg raises with knees bent can help strengthen the lower abs. Lie on your back with knees bent and feet flat on the floor. Lift both legs, keeping the knees bent at a 90-degree angle. Slowly lower the legs back to the floor while maintaining control and keeping the core engaged. Avoid arching the lower back and ensure that the movement is smooth and controlled.

Breath Work and Mindfulness: Breath work is an essential component of core recovery. Practicing deep breathing exercises, focusing on diaphragmatic breathing, can help re-engage the core muscles. Additionally, mindfulness practices, such as yoga or meditation, can promote relaxation and body awareness, helping mothers connect with their core and recognize any discomfort or tension.

Progression and Patience: Rebuilding core strength postpartum is a gradual process that requires patience and consistency. It's important to start with gentle exercises and progress slowly, avoiding highimpact or advanced core exercises until the core is fully healed and strong. Listening to the body and avoiding any exercises that cause pain or discomfort is crucial for safe recovery.

Conclusion: Rebuilding core and abdominal muscles postpartum is a key aspect of physical recovery. Focusing on deep core activation, gentle strengthening exercises, and breath work can help restore core strength and stability. It's important to approach core recovery with patience and mindfulness, ensuring a safe and effective return to physical fitness.

Strengthening the Pelvic Floor

Strengthening the pelvic floor is a crucial aspect of postpartum recovery, as these muscles play a vital role in supporting the pelvic organs, maintaining continence, and contributing to core stability. Pregnancy and childbirth, particularly vaginal delivery, can weaken the pelvic floor, leading to issues such as urinary incontinence, pelvic organ prolapse, and reduced sexual function. Here's a comprehensive guide to understanding and strengthening the pelvic floor postpartum.

Understanding the Pelvic Floor: The pelvic floor is a group of muscles and tissues that form a sling across the pelvis. These muscles support the bladder, uterus, and rectum, and are involved in controlling the release of urine, feces, and gas. During pregnancy, the weight of the growing baby and hormonal changes can weaken the pelvic floor. Vaginal childbirth can further strain these muscles, especially if there is tearing, a prolonged second stage of labor, or the use of instruments like forceps.

Kegel Exercises: Kegel exercises are the most well-known exercise for strengthening the pelvic floor. To perform Kegels, imagine trying to stop the flow of urine midstream, which involves contracting and lifting the pelvic floor muscles. It's important to identify the correct muscles; if you are unsure, try stopping your urine stream once (but do not do this regularly, as it can cause urinary retention). Once the correct muscles are identified, contract them for a count of three to five seconds, then relax for an equal amount of time. Repeat this exercise 10-15 times per session, several times a day. Consistency is key, and results may take a few weeks to become noticeable.

Advanced Pelvic Floor Exercises: As strength improves, more advanced pelvic floor exercises can be introduced. One such exercise is the "elevator" Kegel, where you imagine the pelvic floor muscles as an elevator moving up and down. Gradually contract the muscles to different levels of intensity, holding at each "floor," and then gradually release. Another exercise is the "quick flick," where you quickly contract and release the pelvic floor muscles to improve their responsiveness.

Incorporating Breath Work: Proper breathing is essential during pelvic floor exercises. Diaphragmatic breathing, where the diaphragm expands during inhalation and contracts during exhalation, can help coordinate the pelvic floor muscles with the breath. During the exhale, gently engage the pelvic floor muscles, and relax them during the inhale. This synchronization helps improve muscle control and relaxation.

Pelvic Floor Safe Exercises: While traditional abdominal exercises like crunches can increase intraabdominal pressure and strain the pelvic floor, pelvic floor-safe exercises focus on strengthening the core without this risk. Examples include lying leg lifts, side planks, and exercises on all fours, like the "birddog" exercise. In the bird-dog, start on hands and knees, extend one arm and the opposite leg, hold, and then switch sides. This exercise engages the core and pelvic floor while promoting balance and stability.

Lifestyle Modifications: In addition to exercises, certain lifestyle modifications can help support pelvic floor health. Maintaining a healthy weight reduces pressure on the pelvic floor. Avoiding heavy lifting and practicing proper lifting techniques can prevent further strain. Additionally, managing constipation through a high-fiber diet and staying hydrated can reduce pressure during bowel movements, which can weaken the pelvic floor over time.

When to Seek Professional Help: If pelvic floor weakness persists despite regular exercises, or if there are symptoms such as severe incontinence, pelvic pain, or prolapse, it may be beneficial to consult a pelvic floor physical therapist. These specialists can provide personalized assessment and treatment plans, including biofeedback and manual therapy, to improve pelvic floor function.

Conclusion: Strengthening the pelvic floor is an essential component of postpartum recovery, helping to prevent incontinence, support pelvic organ health, and enhance overall core stability. Kegel exercises, advanced pelvic floor techniques, proper breathing, and pelvic floor-safe exercises are all effective strategies. New mothers should approach pelvic floor strengthening with patience and consistency, and seek professional help if needed to ensure optimal recovery and well-being.

Yoga and Mindfulness Practices

Yoga and mindfulness practices offer a holistic approach to postpartum recovery, addressing physical, emotional, and mental well-being. After childbirth, new mothers often face a range of challenges, including physical discomfort, emotional fluctuations, and the demands of caring for a newborn. Incorporating yoga and mindfulness into the postpartum routine can provide numerous benefits, including improved flexibility, stress reduction, and enhanced emotional balance. Here's an in-depth look at how yoga and mindfulness practices can support postpartum recovery.

Benefits of Yoga Postpartum: Yoga is a gentle form of exercise that combines physical postures (asanas), breath control (pranayama), and meditation. It is particularly beneficial in the postpartum period because it can be adapted to suit individual needs and recovery stages. The physical benefits of yoga include improved flexibility, strength, and posture. Yoga can also help alleviate common postpartum discomforts such as back pain, neck tension, and tight hips. The emphasis on deep breathing and mindfulness in yoga promotes relaxation and stress relief, which can be invaluable for new mothers dealing with the demands of parenting and hormonal changes.

Starting Yoga Postpartum: It's important to consult with a healthcare provider before starting yoga postpartum, especially if there were complications during childbirth. Once cleared for exercise, new mothers can start with gentle, restorative yoga practices. Restorative yoga focuses on passive stretching and relaxation, using props like bolsters, blankets, and blocks to support the body. Poses such as child's pose, cat-cow, and supported reclined butterfly are excellent for gently stretching the back, hips, and chest, and can be soothing for both body and mind.

Core and Pelvic Floor Integration: Postpartum yoga can also help with core and pelvic floor recovery. Specific poses and breathing techniques can aid in re-engaging these muscles safely. For example, the "bridge" pose helps strengthen the glutes, lower back, and core. In this pose, the mother lies on her back with knees bent and feet flat on the floor, lifting the hips while engaging the core and pelvic floor. The "happy baby" pose, where one lies on the back and holds the feet with knees bent and wide, can gently stretch the pelvic floor and inner thighs, promoting relaxation and flexibility.

Mindfulness and Meditation: Mindfulness and meditation are integral components of yoga that focus on cultivating present-moment awareness and emotional regulation. Postpartum, these practices can help new mothers manage stress, anxiety, and the emotional ups and downs that often accompany the transition to parenthood. Mindfulness involves paying attention to the present moment without judgment, which can be practiced during yoga or in daily activities. Simple mindfulness exercises include focusing on the breath, practicing gratitude, or performing a body scan to notice sensations and tension areas.

Breathwork (Pranayama): Breathwork, or pranayama, is a key aspect of yoga that involves conscious control of the breath. Deep breathing exercises can help calm the nervous system, reduce stress, and improve oxygenation. One effective technique is "ujjayi" or "ocean breath," where one inhales deeply through the nose, then exhales slowly while slightly constricting the back of the throat, creating a soft ocean-like sound. This technique can be calming and help maintain focus during yoga practice or stressful moments.

Incorporating Baby into Practice: Postpartum yoga can also be a bonding experience when incorporating the baby into the practice. "Mom and baby" yoga classes offer poses and movements that include the baby, creating a nurturing environment for physical activity and emotional connection. Gentle movements, such as rocking and swaying, can soothe the baby while the mother performs yoga poses. This shared practice can strengthen the mother-infant bond and provide a playful and enjoyable way to exercise.

CHAPTER 7: POSTPARTUM BODY IMAGE AND SELFESTEEM

Navigating Body Changes

The postpartum period brings significant changes to a woman's body, often in ways that can be surprising and challenging. Understanding and navigating these changes is crucial for both physical recovery and emotional well-being. After pregnancy and childbirth, women may experience shifts in weight, shape, and function, all of which are part of the natural process of adapting to the needs of motherhood.

Physical Changes: During pregnancy, the body undergoes numerous transformations, including weight gain, skin stretching, and hormonal fluctuations. Postpartum, the process of "snapping back" is not immediate and can take time. Common physical changes include a soft and expanded abdomen due to stretched abdominal muscles and skin, which may also show signs of diastasis recti (separation of the abdominal muscles). Breasts may be fuller or feel engorged, especially if breastfeeding, and the skin might exhibit stretch marks, particularly on the stomach, breasts, thighs, and hips.

Another notable change is the redistribution of body fat. While some women may lose weight relatively quickly, others may retain some of the fat stores that were naturally accumulated during pregnancy. This fat distribution can sometimes shift, with some areas, such as the hips and thighs, retaining more weight. This is a normal part of the body's adaptation to support the demands of motherhood, including breastfeeding.

Emotional Response to Changes: The emotional response to postpartum body changes varies widely among women. While some may feel empowered and proud of their body's ability to create and sustain life, others may struggle with the alterations in their appearance. This can be especially true in a society that often idealizes slim and toned bodies, making it difficult for new mothers to accept and love their postpartum figures. The pressure to quickly return to a pre-pregnancy body can lead to feelings of inadequacy, frustration, and even depression.

Acceptance and Adaptation: Adapting to these changes involves a process of acceptance and understanding that the postpartum body is a testament to the incredible process of bringing a new life into the world. It's important for new mothers to recognize that recovery and body changes are part of a natural journey, and each woman's experience is unique. There is no standard timeline or ideal postpartum body, and it's crucial to focus on health and well-being rather than striving for an unrealistic ideal.

Practical Strategies: Practically, navigating these changes can involve a variety of approaches. Engaging in gentle postpartum exercises, such as walking, yoga, or Pilates, can help women feel more connected to their bodies and aid in physical recovery. It's also important to maintain a balanced diet that supports healing and overall health, rather than restrictive dieting, which can be harmful both physically and emotionally.

Self-Care and Compassion: Self-care practices are essential during this period. This can include prioritizing rest, seeking support from partners, family, or friends, and setting aside time for activities that bring joy and relaxation. Practicing self-compassion and kindness towards oneself is critical. Acknowledging that body changes are a normal and expected part of the postpartum journey can help in fostering a positive outlook.

Conclusion: Navigating body changes postpartum is a multifaceted experience that involves physical adaptation and emotional resilience. It's a time that calls for self-compassion, realistic expectations, and a focus on health and well-being. By embracing these changes and understanding that they are a part of the incredible journey of motherhood, new mothers can navigate this transition with greater ease and confidence.

Building Positive Body Image

Building a positive body image postpartum is an essential component of mental and emotional well-being. After the transformative experience of pregnancy and childbirth, women often face a new relationship with their bodies. This period requires a shift in perspective, focusing on self-acceptance and appreciation rather than societal standards of beauty. Developing a positive body image involves acknowledging and valuing the incredible capabilities of the body, practicing self-compassion, and challenging negative thoughts and perceptions.

Understanding Body Image: Body image refers to the perceptions, thoughts, and feelings a person has about their physical appearance. For new mothers, body image can be particularly vulnerable due to the significant changes their bodies undergo during pregnancy and postpartum. Media portrayals of "ideal" postpartum bodies can exacerbate these challenges, often presenting unrealistic images that do not reflect the diversity of postpartum experiences.

The Role of Media and Society: The media often promotes an idealized image of slim, toned postpartum bodies, which can lead to unrealistic expectations and self-criticism. It's important for new mothers to recognize that these representations are often not accurate or achievable for most women. Social media, while offering a platform for sharing experiences, can also contribute to comparison and feelings of inadequacy. Curating a positive social media feed that includes diverse and body-positive content can help counteract these pressures.

Strategies for Building Positive Body Image: Developing a positive body image involves several strategies. Firstly, practicing gratitude for the body's abilities is crucial. Acknowledging the physical and emotional strength required to go through pregnancy and childbirth can foster appreciation for the body's capabilities. This mindset shift from focusing on appearance to recognizing functionality can be liberating. Self-compassion is another key component. New mothers should treat themselves with the same kindness and understanding they would offer a friend. This includes acknowledging that it's normal to have mixed feelings about body changes and that it's okay to take time to adjust.

Challenging Negative Thoughts: Cognitive-behavioral techniques can be useful in challenging negative thoughts and beliefs about body image. For example, when negative thoughts arise, such as "I should look a certain way," it's helpful to question these beliefs and replace them with more realistic and positive affirmations. Statements like "My body is strong and capable" or "I am more than my appearance" can help shift focus away from unrealistic ideals.

Support Systems and Communication: Building a positive body image is not solely an individual effort; support systems play a crucial role. Open communication with partners, family, and friends about body image concerns can provide emotional support and understanding. Surrounding oneself with supportive and body-positive individuals can reinforce positive self-perception and reduce the impact of negative societal messages.

The Role of Fashion and Self-Expression: Fashion can also play a role in fostering a positive body image. Wearing clothes that are comfortable and make new mothers feel good about themselves can enhance self-confidence. It's important to choose clothing that fits well and accommodates the body's changes rather than attempting to fit into pre-pregnancy clothes prematurely. Embracing new styles and finding joy in self-expression through fashion can be an empowering experience.

Mindfulness and Self-Acceptance: Mindfulness practices can aid in developing a positive body image by encouraging present-moment awareness and acceptance. Mindful meditation, focusing on body sensations without judgment, can help cultivate a neutral or positive relationship with the body. Accepting the current state of the body as it is, without striving for perfection, is a powerful step towards body positivity.

Fashion and Comfort Tips

The postpartum period brings a unique set of challenges and changes, and finding fashion and comfort tips that work can significantly boost a new mother's confidence and ease. The focus during this time should be on clothing that is not only practical and comfortable but also helps new mothers feel good about themselves as they navigate their new roles. Here are some essential fashion and comfort tips tailored to the postpartum experience.

Comfort is Key: In the postpartum phase, comfort becomes paramount. The body is still healing, and new mothers may experience physical discomforts, such as swelling, soreness, or engorgement. Soft, breathable fabrics like cotton or bamboo are ideal as they are gentle on the skin and allow for breathability. Elastic waistbands and loose-fitting clothing provide comfort and flexibility, accommodating changes in body shape and size.

Supportive Undergarments: Investing in good quality, supportive undergarments is crucial. Nursing bras, which provide easy access for breastfeeding and sufficient support for engorged breasts, are a musthave. Look for bras with adjustable straps and multiple hook options to accommodate size changes. Highwaisted underwear can offer gentle support to the abdomen and are particularly beneficial for those recovering from a cesarean section, as they avoid irritating the incision area.

Functional Fashion: Postpartum fashion should prioritize functionality, especially for breastfeeding mothers. Nursing tops and dresses with easy access panels or buttons make breastfeeding more convenient. Layering is another practical strategy; wearing a nursing tank underneath a regular top allows for discreet breastfeeding. Wrap dresses and tops are not only stylish but also functional, providing easy access for nursing while flattering the changing figure.

Maternity and Postpartum Wear: Many maternity clothes are designed to be worn during both pregnancy and postpartum, making them a versatile investment. Maternity leggings, for example, often feature a high, stretchy waistband that can provide support to the postpartum belly. Tunics, maxi dresses, and empire-waist tops are also excellent choices as they offer comfort, style, and room for the body's changes.

Choosing the Right Footwear: Footwear is another important consideration postpartum, as feet may still be swollen or require extra support. Comfortable shoes with good arch support can help alleviate any back or foot pain, common postpartum complaints. Slip-on styles can be particularly convenient when holding a baby or carrying multiple items.

Clothing for Body Confidence: Feeling good in what you wear can significantly impact your mood and self-esteem. While comfort is essential, incorporating elements of style that align with personal preferences can enhance body confidence. Choosing colors, patterns, and styles that you love can uplift your spirits. For example, a bright scarf, a favorite pair of earrings, or a comfortable yet stylish cardigan can add a touch of joy to an everyday outfit.

Loungewear and Pajamas: As much of the postpartum period involves time spent at home, comfortable loungewear and pajamas are vital. Look for sets that are cozy yet presentable enough to wear throughout the day, making it easy to transition from sleeping to caring for the baby without feeling underdressed. Button-up pajama tops or nursing nightgowns are practical for nighttime feedings.

Caring for the New Body: Along with choosing the right clothing, taking care of the postpartum body is essential. Moisturizing the skin, particularly areas like the belly and breasts, can help with elasticity and comfort. Staying hydrated and eating a balanced diet also contributes to overall well-being and can affect how one feels in their clothes.

Adapting to Seasonal Changes: Depending on the season, postpartum fashion needs may vary. In colder months, layering is key—consider warm, stretchy leggings, oversized sweaters, and shawls. In warmer weather, light, breathable fabrics, and flowy dresses can provide comfort. Always consider the practicality of the clothing in relation to caring for a newborn, ensuring ease of movement and temperature regulation.

Reconnecting with Your Partner Intimately

Reconnecting with a partner intimately after childbirth can be a delicate process, involving physical, emotional, and psychological dimensions. The postpartum period brings significant changes, and it's natural for couples to experience shifts in their relationship dynamics. Understanding the nuances of this transition and approaching it with patience, communication, and empathy is key to reestablishing intimacy.

Physical Recovery and Readiness: The physical recovery process after childbirth varies from woman to woman. Whether the delivery was vaginal or via cesarean section, the body needs time to heal. For vaginal births, it is generally recommended to wait until postpartum bleeding has stopped, and any tears or episiotomies have healed before resuming sexual activity. This usually takes about six weeks, but the timeframe can vary. For cesarean deliveries, healing the surgical incision and ensuring overall physical recovery are essential.

During this time, many women may experience vaginal dryness, especially if breastfeeding, due to hormonal changes. Using water-based lubricants can help alleviate discomfort. It's also common for the pelvic floor muscles to feel weakened, which can impact the experience of intercourse. Kegel exercises can help strengthen these muscles and improve control.

Emotional and Psychological Considerations: Beyond the physical aspects, emotional and psychological readiness plays a crucial role in resuming intimate activities. The postpartum period is often marked by hormonal fluctuations, sleep deprivation, and the demands of caring for a newborn. These factors can lead to feelings of fatigue, stress, and sometimes, a decreased interest in sex. It's important for both partners to understand that a reduced libido is normal and does not reflect a lack of love or attraction.

Communication is vital in navigating these changes. Couples should openly discuss their feelings, desires, and any concerns they may have. This includes talking about any fears or discomforts related to physical intimacy. For the partner who did not give birth, it's important to be supportive and understanding, recognizing that their partner may need time and space to feel ready for intimacy.

Rebuilding Emotional Intimacy: Emotional intimacy is a cornerstone of a healthy relationship and can be especially important during the postpartum period. Reconnecting emotionally can involve spending quality time together, even if it's just a few quiet moments after the baby goes to sleep. Acts of kindness, sharing responsibilities, and expressing appreciation for each other can strengthen the emotional bond. Physical touch, such as holding hands, hugging, or cuddling, can also help maintain a sense of closeness. These small gestures can be comforting and reassuring, helping to bridge the gap as the couple transitions back to sexual intimacy.

Exploring New Forms of Intimacy: It's important to recognize that intimacy is not limited to sexual activity. During the postpartum period, couples can explore other ways to connect, such as through affectionate gestures, deep conversations, or shared hobbies. This period can also be a time to rediscover each other's non-sexual love languages, whether it's through words of affirmation, acts of service, or spending quality time together.

For some couples, seeking new ways to be intimate might include exploring different forms of physical closeness, like massage, which can be both relaxing and intimate. Experimenting with different types of touch and communication can help rekindle the connection.

Seeking Professional Support: If resuming intimacy proves to be challenging or if there are unresolved issues, it may be helpful to seek professional support. A couple therapist or sex therapist can provide a safe space to explore concerns, improve communication, and find solutions that work for both partners. This can be particularly beneficial if there are underlying issues such as postpartum depression or anxiety, which can affect intimacy.

Patience and Compassion: Above all, patience and compassion are essential. Reconnecting intimately after childbirth is a gradual process, and it's important to set realistic expectations. Both partners should approach this transition with an open mind and a willingness to understand each other's needs and boundaries. Remembering that this is a time of significant change and that adjustments are normal can help alleviate pressure.

CHAPTER 8: SLEEP AND REST

Understanding Postpartum Sleep Deprivation

Postpartum sleep deprivation is a widespread issue affecting new parents, especially mothers, in the early weeks and months following childbirth. Understanding this phenomenon involves recognizing its causes, impacts, and ways to address it to support better recovery and well-being during this transformative period.

Causes of Postpartum Sleep Deprivation: Sleep deprivation in the postpartum period primarily stems from the demands of caring for a newborn. Newborns typically sleep in short bursts, waking every few hours for feeding, diaper changes, and comfort. This fragmented sleep pattern significantly disrupts parents' sleep cycles, leading to chronic sleep deficits. Additionally, the stress of adjusting to a new routine, combined with physical recovery from childbirth, can make it harder for parents to get restorative sleep. Hormonal changes after childbirth can also play a role in sleep disturbances. Fluctuations in hormones such as estrogen and progesterone can affect sleep patterns, making it difficult for new mothers to fall asleep or stay asleep even when the baby is resting. Sleep disorders like insomnia or sleep apnea may also be exacerbated during this period.

Impact on Physical Health: Sleep deprivation can have profound effects on physical health. The body's ability to heal from childbirth is compromised when it lacks adequate rest. This can lead to prolonged recovery times and increased susceptibility to infections. Chronic sleep deprivation also weakens the immune system, making it harder to fend off illnesses.

Impact on Mental Health: The emotional and psychological impact of sleep deprivation is equally significant. Fatigue can lead to mood swings, irritability, and heightened stress levels. For some new mothers, this can contribute to or exacerbate postpartum depression and anxiety. Sleep deprivation impairs cognitive functions such as memory, decision-making, and concentration, which can further compound feelings of overwhelm and inadequacy.

Long-Term Consequences: Persistent sleep deprivation can have long-term consequences for both parents and their relationship with their baby. It can strain interpersonal relationships, affect parenting quality, and diminish overall quality of life. Addressing sleep deprivation early on is crucial to prevent these long-term effects and support better overall well-being.

Tips for Better Sleep and Rest

Achieving better sleep and rest during the postpartum period can be challenging but is essential for overall well-being and recovery. Implementing practical strategies can help new parents make the most of the sleep opportunities available and improve their quality of rest.

Prioritize Sleep: One of the most effective strategies for better sleep is to prioritize it whenever possible. This may involve adjusting daily routines to ensure that sleep takes precedence. New parents should consider delegating non-essential tasks and focusing on resting during the baby's sleep periods. Recognizing that rest is crucial for recovery can help alleviate feelings of guilt associated with taking time for oneself.

Create a Relaxing Sleep Environment: A conducive sleep environment is vital for improving sleep quality. This includes keeping the bedroom cool, dark, and quiet. Investing in blackout curtains, a white noise machine, or a fan can help create a calming atmosphere conducive to sleep. For the baby, establishing a safe and comfortable sleep space with a firm mattress and minimal distractions can support better sleep patterns.

Establish a Routine: Developing a consistent bedtime routine can help signal to both parents and the baby that it is time to wind down. This routine might include calming activities such as reading a book, taking a warm bath, or practicing relaxation techniques. Consistency in bedtime routines can help both parents and the baby transition into a more relaxed state and improve overall sleep quality.

Share Nighttime Responsibilities: Sharing nighttime responsibilities between partners or caregivers can significantly alleviate the burden of sleep deprivation. For breastfeeding mothers, this might involve pumping breast milk in advance so that the partner can handle one or more nighttime feedings. Alternatively, partners can assist with diaper changes, soothing the baby, or other nighttime tasks to allow the mother to get more uninterrupted rest.

Limit Stimulants and Screen Time: Avoiding stimulants such as caffeine and nicotine, especially in the late afternoon and evening, can help improve sleep quality. Additionally, limiting screen time before bed can support better sleep. The blue light emitted by phones, tablets, and computers can interfere with the production of melatonin, the hormone that regulates sleep. Opt for relaxing activities that do not involve screens to help prepare the body for sleep.

Practice Relaxation Techniques: Incorporating relaxation techniques into the bedtime routine can enhance sleep quality. Techniques such as deep breathing, progressive muscle relaxation, or gentle stretching can help calm the mind and prepare the body for rest. Even a few minutes of focused relaxation can make a significant difference in how easily one falls asleep and how restful the sleep is.

Napping Strategically: Napping during the day can help compensate for lost nighttime sleep. Short naps of 20 to 30 minutes can be refreshing and improve alertness without interfering with nighttime sleep. Longer naps, if necessary, should be timed earlier in the day to prevent disrupting the ability to fall asleep at night. Coordinating nap times with the baby's sleep schedule can also help maximize rest.

Seek Support: Don't hesitate to seek support from family, friends, or a professional if sleep deprivation becomes overwhelming. Accepting offers of help with household tasks, meal preparation, or baby care can free up time for rest. Additionally, consulting a healthcare provider for advice on managing sleep difficulties or addressing underlying issues can provide valuable guidance and support.

The Role of Napping

Napping is a critical strategy for managing sleep deprivation and supporting recovery during the postpartum period. Understanding the benefits and best practices for napping can help new parents make the most of these short periods of rest and enhance their overall well-being.

Benefits of Napping: Napping provides several benefits for new parents. It helps mitigate the effects of sleep deprivation by offering an opportunity to catch up on lost sleep. Even brief naps can improve mood, reduce fatigue, and enhance cognitive functioning. For mothers recovering from childbirth, napping supports physical recovery by allowing the body to heal and replenish energy levels.

Timing and Duration: The timing and duration of naps can significantly impact their effectiveness. Short naps of 20 to 30 minutes are ideal for a quick refresh, improving alertness and mood without leading to sleep inertia—a groggy feeling that can occur after longer naps. These short naps can help parents stay energized and manage the demands of caring for a newborn.

Longer naps, lasting 60 to 90 minutes, allow the body to complete a full sleep cycle, including deep sleep stages. This can be more restorative but requires careful timing to avoid interfering with nighttime sleep. It is best to take longer naps earlier in the day to prevent them from disrupting the ability to fall asleep at night.

Creating an Ideal Napping Environment: An ideal napping environment is crucial for maximizing rest. This includes a quiet, dark, and comfortable space where interruptions are minimized. Using blackout curtains, a white noise machine, or an eye mask can help create a conducive environment for napping. For parents, having a comfortable place to lie down and relax is essential for making the most of napping opportunities.

Overcoming Barriers: Some new parents may face barriers to napping, such as anxiety, stress, or a sense of needing to be constantly alert. It is important to recognize that napping is a necessary part of postpartum recovery and well-being. To overcome these barriers, parents can set a regular nap schedule, even if the actual nap times vary. Consistency in trying to rest when the baby sleeps can help the body adapt and make the most of available rest periods.

Managing Expectations: It is important to manage expectations regarding napping during the postpartum period. While napping can significantly improve rest and recovery, it may not be possible to achieve uninterrupted or ideal nap times every day. Being flexible and adapting to the baby's schedule can help reduce stress and improve the overall effectiveness of napping.

Combining Naps with Other Strategies: Combining napping with other sleep strategies can enhance overall rest and well-being. This includes prioritizing sleep during the night, sharing nighttime responsibilities with a partner, and creating a relaxing sleep environment. Integrating napping into a broader sleep strategy can help parents manage sleep deprivation more effectively and support better overall recovery.

Strategies for Managing Nighttime Feedings

Managing nighttime feedings effectively is crucial for new parents, particularly those who are breastfeeding. Implementing strategies to handle these feedings can help alleviate some of the stress and disruption associated with nighttime care and support better sleep for both parents and the baby. **Establish a Nighttime Routine**: Creating a consistent nighttime feeding routine can help both parents and the baby adjust to nighttime care. Establishing a calming pre-feeding routine, such as dimming the lights, playing soft music, or reading a short story, can signal that it's time for sleep. This routine can help the baby wind down and make the transition between wakefulness and sleep smoother.

Optimize Feedings: Ensuring that the baby is well-fed before going to sleep can help extend the duration of sleep between feedings. For breastfeeding mothers, this might involve offering both breasts during a feeding session to ensure the baby gets a full feed. For bottle-feeding, making sure the baby consumes a sufficient amount of milk can reduce the likelihood of waking up due to hunger.

Use a Nightlight and Minimize Disruptions: Keeping the environment calm and low-light during nighttime feedings can help both the baby and Parents transition back to sleep more easily. Using a soft nightlight instead of bright overhead lights can create a soothing atmosphere without fully waking either the baby or the mother. Minimizing noise and keeping interactions brief can also help maintain a sleepconducive environment.

Share Responsibilities: Sharing nighttime feeding responsibilities with a partner or caregiver can significantly alleviate the burden of sleep deprivation. For breastfeeding mothers, this might involve pumping breast milk ahead of time so that the partner can handle one or more nighttime feedings. Partners can also assist with diaper changes, soothing the baby, or other nighttime tasks to allow the mother to get more uninterrupted rest.

Prepare for Nighttime Feedings: Having everything needed for nighttime feedings readily accessible can streamline the process and minimize disruptions. Preparing bottles in advance, keeping a supply of clean burp cloths, and having a comfortable feeding area set up can make nighttime care more efficient. For breastfeeding mothers, having a water bottle, snacks, and a comfortable pillow within reach can make feedings more convenient.

Track Feedings and Sleep Patterns: Keeping track of the baby's feeding and sleep patterns can help identify any trends or issues. This information can be useful for adjusting feeding routines and understanding the baby's needs. There are various apps and journals available that can assist with tracking and managing nighttime feedings.

Practice Self-Care: Managing nighttime feedings effectively also involves taking care of oneself. Ensuring that both parents are getting adequate rest during the day, if possible, can help mitigate the effects of nighttime disruptions. Practicing self-care, such as relaxation techniques, seeking support from friends and family, or engaging in activities that help manage stress, can also help improve the overall experience of nighttime care.

Be Flexible and Adapt: Flexibility is key when managing nighttime feedings. Babies' sleep patterns can change frequently, and what works one night may not work the next. Being adaptable and willing to adjust strategies as needed can help reduce stress and improve the overall experience of nighttime care.

CHAPTER 9: POSTPARTUM COMPLICATIONS

Recognizing Signs of Infection

Postpartum infections can pose serious health risks for new mothers, making early recognition and prompt treatment crucial for recovery and overall well-being. Understanding the signs and symptoms of postpartum infections helps new mothers seek timely medical attention and prevent complications. **Types of Postpartum Infections**: Postpartum infections can affect various areas of the body, including the uterus, breasts, and surgical sites if a cesarean section was performed. Common types include endometritis (infection of the uterine lining), mastitis (breast infection), and wound infections from a cesarean section or episiotomy.

Signs of Endometritis: Endometritis often presents with symptoms such as fever, abdominal pain, and abnormal vaginal discharge. The discharge may be foul-smelling and can vary in color from yellow to green. Women may also experience chills, rapid heart rate, and a general feeling of illness. If these symptoms are observed, it is essential to consult a healthcare provider for evaluation and treatment. **Signs of Mastitis**: Mastitis typically affects one breast and can cause symptoms such as redness, swelling, and warmth in the breast tissue. The affected area may be tender or painful, and there may be flu-like symptoms such as fever, chills, and body aches. Mastitis can result from blocked milk ducts or bacterial infection and often requires antibiotic treatment and proper breastfeeding management.

Signs of Wound Infection: Infections at the site of a cesarean section or episiotomy can manifest as redness, swelling, increased pain, or drainage of pus from the wound. The area may also feel warm to the touch. Systemic symptoms like fever and chills can accompany wound infections. Prompt medical attention is necessary to address wound infections effectively and prevent further complications. **Preventive Measures**: Preventing postpartum infections involves practicing good hygiene, including frequent handwashing and proper care of the wound site. For breastfeeding mothers, ensuring proper latch and hygiene during feedings can help prevent mastitis. Additionally, staying hydrated, maintaining a healthy diet, and following post-surgical care instructions can support the body's natural defenses against infection.

Managing Postpartum Hemorrhage

Postpartum hemorrhage (PPH) is a serious complication that can occur after childbirth and requires immediate attention to ensure maternal safety. Understanding its signs, causes, and management strategies is essential for effective treatment and recovery.

Defining Postpartum Hemorrhage: Postpartum hemorrhage is defined as excessive bleeding after the delivery of the baby. It is typically classified into two categories: early (or primary) postpartum hemorrhage, which occurs within the first 24 hours after childbirth, and late (or secondary) postpartum hemorrhage, which occurs between 24 hours and 12 weeks after delivery.

Signs and Symptoms: Key signs of postpartum hemorrhage include excessive vaginal bleeding, which may be heavier than a normal menstrual period, or the passage of large blood clots. Other symptoms may include rapid heart rate, low blood pressure, and signs of shock, such as dizziness, weakness, or confusion. Monitoring the amount and nature of vaginal bleeding is crucial in identifying potential hemorrhage.

Causes of Postpartum Hemorrhage: The primary causes of postpartum hemorrhage include uterine atony (lack of uterine muscle tone), retained placental fragments, and lacerations in the birth canal. Uterine atony is the most common cause and occurs when the uterus fails to contract effectively after delivery. Retained placental fragments can prevent the uterus from contracting properly, leading to continued bleeding.

Management Strategies: Effective management of postpartum hemorrhage involves prompt intervention to control bleeding and stabilize the patient. Immediate actions may include:

- **Uterine Massage and Medication**: Fundal massage and administration of uterotonics, such as oxytocin, can help stimulate uterine contractions and reduce bleeding. Uterotonics are medications that help the uterus contract and expel any retained placenta.

- **Manual Removal of Retained Placenta**: If retained placental fragments are identified, manual removal may be necessary. This procedure is performed by a healthcare provider to ensure complete expulsion of the placenta and reduce the risk of continued bleeding.

- **Surgical Intervention**: In severe cases of postpartum hemorrhage, surgical intervention may be required. This may include procedures such as dilation and curettage (D&C) to remove retained placenta or repair lacerations.

- **Blood Transfusion**: If significant blood loss occurs, a blood transfusion may be necessary to restore blood volume and stabilize the patient.

Monitoring and Follow-Up: Continuous monitoring of vital signs, bleeding, and uterine tone is essential during the immediate postpartum period. Healthcare providers will assess the effectiveness of interventions and make any necessary adjustments to ensure optimal recovery.

Blood Clots and Deep Vein Thrombosis (DVT)

Blood clots and deep vein thrombosis (DVT) are potential complications in the postpartum period that require careful management to prevent serious health issues. Understanding their signs, risk factors, and management strategies is crucial for maintaining maternal health and safety.

Understanding DVT: Deep vein thrombosis (DVT) refers to the formation of a blood clot in a deep vein, typically in the legs. It can lead to serious complications, including pulmonary embolism, if the clot dislodges and travels to the lungs. Postpartum women are at increased risk for DVT due to changes in blood clotting and reduced mobility during the recovery period.

Signs and Symptoms of DVT: Common signs of DVT include swelling, redness, and warmth in the affected leg. The leg may feel painful or tender, and there may be noticeable swelling, particularly in the calf. In some cases, the symptoms may be mild or not immediately apparent, making it important to be vigilant for any changes in leg comfort or appearance.

Risk Factors: Several factors can increase the risk of developing DVT during the postpartum period. These include:

- **Prolonged Bed Rest**: Extended periods of immobility, such as during recovery from a cesarean section, can contribute to blood clot formation. Moving and stretching the legs regularly can help reduce this risk.

- **Hormonal Changes**: Postpartum hormonal changes can affect blood clotting, increasing the likelihood of clot formation. Women who have a history of blood clotting disorders may be at higher risk.

- **Obesity and Smoking**: Excess weight and smoking are additional risk factors that can contribute to the development of DVT. Maintaining a healthy weight and avoiding smoking can help mitigate these risks.

Prevention and Management: Preventing and managing DVT involves several strategies:

- **Regular Movement**: Encouraging regular movement and leg exercises can help improve circulation and reduce the risk of clot formation. Simple activities such as ankle circles, leg raises, and walking can be beneficial.

- **Compression Stockings**: Wearing compression stockings can help improve blood flow in the legs and reduce the risk of DVT. These stockings apply gentle pressure to the legs, aiding circulation and preventing clot formation.

- **Medication**: In some cases, healthcare providers may prescribe anticoagulant medications to reduce the risk of blood clots. These medications help prevent clot formation and may be recommended based on individual risk factors and medical history.
- **Monitoring and Evaluation**: If DVT is suspected, healthcare providers will conduct a thorough evaluation, which may include imaging tests such as ultrasound to confirm the presence of a blood clot. Treatment may involve medications to dissolve the clot and prevent further complications.

Postpartum Thyroiditis and Hormonal Imbalances

Postpartum thyroiditis and hormonal imbalances are conditions that can affect new mothers, impacting their physical and emotional well-being. Understanding these issues, their symptoms, and management strategies is essential for maintaining health during the postpartum period.

Postpartum Thyroiditis: Postpartum thyroiditis is an inflammation of the thyroid gland that occurs within the first year after childbirth. It can lead to either hyperthyroidism (overactive thyroid) or hypothyroidism (underactive thyroid). The condition may be transient or persist beyond the postpartum period.

Symptoms of Postpartum Thyroiditis: Symptoms can vary depending on whether the thyroiditis presents as hyperthyroidism or hypothyroidism. Hyperthyroidism may cause symptoms such as rapid heart rate, weight loss, anxiety, and heat intolerance. Hypothyroidism, on the other hand, can lead to symptoms such as fatigue, weight gain, depression, and cold intolerance. In some cases, postpartum thyroiditis may be asymptomatic or present with mild symptoms that are easily overlooked.

Diagnosis and Management: Diagnosis of postpartum thyroiditis involves blood tests to measure thyroid hormone levels and assess thyroid function. Treatment may vary depending on the type and severity of thyroid dysfunction:

- **Hyperthyroidism**: Treatment for hyperthyroidism may include medications to regulate thyroid hormone levels and manage symptoms. In some cases, beta-blockers may be prescribed to control symptoms such as rapid heart rate and anxiety.
- **Hypothyroidism**: Treatment for hypothyroidism typically involves thyroid hormone replacement therapy. Medications such as levothyroxine are used to normalize thyroid hormone levels and alleviate symptoms.

Hormonal Imbalances: Postpartum hormonal imbalances are common and can affect mood, energy levels, and overall well-being. Hormonal changes after childbirth can lead to fluctuations in estrogen, progesterone, and other hormones, impacting various aspects of health.

Symptoms of Hormonal Imbalances: Symptoms may include mood swings, fatigue, difficulty sleeping, and changes in menstrual cycles. Women may also experience symptoms related to estrogen deficiency, such as hot flashes, vaginal dryness, and decreased libido. Hormonal imbalances can also contribute to postpartum depression and anxiety.

Management Strategies: Managing hormonal imbalances involves addressing underlying issues and supporting overall health:

- **Balanced Diet**: A nutritious diet rich in vitamins and minerals can help support hormonal balance. Foods rich in omega-3 fatty acids, calcium, and vitamin D are beneficial for overall health.
- **Regular Exercise**: Engaging in regular physical activity can help regulate hormones, improve mood, and support overall well-being. Exercise also promotes better sleep and reduces stress.
- **Stress Management**: Managing stress through relaxation techniques, mindfulness, and support from loved ones can help alleviate symptoms of hormonal imbalances. Finding time for self-care and relaxation is essential for maintaining balance.

Other Potential Complications

In addition to the common postpartum complications mentioned, several other issues may arise during the postpartum period, requiring awareness and appropriate management. Understanding these potential complications helps ensure comprehensive care and support for new mothers.

Urinary Incontinence: Urinary incontinence, or the involuntary leakage of urine, is a common issue following childbirth. It can occur due to the stretching and weakening of pelvic floor muscles during pregnancy and delivery. Women may experience leakage when coughing, sneezing, or laughing. Management strategies include pelvic floor exercises (Kegels), physical therapy, and behavioral techniques to improve bladder control.

Perineal Pain: Pain in the perineal area, which includes the tissues between the vaginal opening and the anus, is common after vaginal delivery. This pain can result from tearing, episiotomy, or general trauma during childbirth. Managing perineal pain involves proper wound care, using ice packs, taking sitz baths, and using over-the-counter pain medications as needed.

Diastasis Recti: Diastasis recti is a condition in which the abdominal muscles separate during pregnancy, leading to a protruding abdomen and weakened core. This condition can affect physical function and selfesteem. Treatment typically involves physical therapy focused on strengthening the abdominal muscles and improving core stability.

Postpartum Headaches: Postpartum headaches can be caused by various factors, including hormonal changes, dehydration, or tension. In some cases, headaches may be related to high blood pressure or preeclampsia. Managing postpartum headaches involves staying hydrated, getting adequate rest, and addressing any underlying conditions with medical guidance.

Gastrointestinal Issues: Gastrointestinal problems, such as constipation or hemorrhoids, are common after childbirth. Constipation can result from changes in diet, reduced physical activity, or pain medications. Hemorrhoids may occur due to increased pressure during pregnancy and delivery. Managing these issues involves maintaining a high-fiber diet, staying hydrated, and using over-the-counter remedies as needed.

CHAPTER 10: POSTPARTUM RELATIONSHIPS AND SOCIAL SUPPORT

Adjusting to Parenthood

Becoming a parent marks a profound transition in life, often accompanied by a mix of joy, excitement, and challenges. The adjustment to parenthood involves navigating new responsibilities, changing routines, and evolving roles within the family. Understanding these changes and finding ways to manage them effectively is key to a smooth transition and maintaining family harmony.

The New Dynamic: The arrival of a baby brings significant changes to family dynamics. Parents must adapt to new routines that revolve around the baby's needs, including feeding, sleeping, and diapering. This adjustment can be overwhelming as parents learn to balance their new responsibilities with their existing roles and relationships. It's normal to experience a period of adaptation as everyone finds their rhythm.

Emotional Adjustments: The emotional impact of becoming a parent can be profound. New parents may experience a wide range of emotions, including joy, anxiety, and even sadness. Hormonal changes, lack of sleep, and the sheer responsibility of caring for a newborn can contribute to emotional fluctuations. Open communication between partners and seeking emotional support can help manage these changes and maintain emotional well-being.

Time Management: Managing time becomes crucial when adjusting to parenthood. New parents often find themselves juggling baby care with household responsibilities and personal needs. Establishing a routine can help bring structure to the day, but flexibility is also important. Prioritizing tasks, delegating responsibilities, and using time management tools can help parents navigate their new schedules more effectively.

Support and Self-Care: Seeking support from family, friends, or professional services can ease the transition to parenthood. Taking time for self-care is equally important. This might involve short breaks, pursuing hobbies, or simply finding moments of relaxation. Prioritizing self-care helps parents stay healthy and energized, which benefits both their well-being and their ability to care for their baby. **Professional Guidance**: Many new parents benefit from professional guidance, such as counseling or parenting classes. These resources can offer valuable advice on parenting strategies, stress management, and coping with the challenges of parenthood. Seeking help from experts can provide reassurance and practical tools for adjusting to the new roles and responsibilities.

Strengthening the Couple's Relationship

The arrival of a baby can impact a couple's relationship in various ways. Strengthening the relationship amid the demands of parenthood is crucial for maintaining a healthy and supportive partnership. Effective communication, shared responsibilities, and intentional quality time are key elements in nurturing the couple's bond during this transitional period.

Communication: Open and honest communication is vital for maintaining a strong relationship. New parents should make time to discuss their feelings, concerns, and expectations. Sharing experiences and being receptive to each other's needs helps prevent misunderstandings and fosters a supportive environment. Regular check-ins and discussing challenges can help couples stay connected and address any issues before they escalate.

Shared Responsibilities: Dividing parenting and household responsibilities equitably can help reduce stress and prevent feelings of resentment. Both partners should actively participate in caring for the baby, managing household tasks, and supporting each other. Establishing clear roles and being flexible in adjusting these roles as needed can contribute to a balanced partnership.

Quality Time: Finding moments to spend quality time together is essential for strengthening the couple's relationship. While the demands of a newborn can make it challenging to find time for each other, even small gestures can make a difference. Simple activities, such as having a meal together, taking short walks, or watching a movie, can help couples reconnect and maintain their bond.

Expressing Appreciation: Showing appreciation and acknowledging each other's efforts can strengthen the relationship. Expressing gratitude for support, recognizing each other's contributions, and offering words of encouragement can foster a positive and loving atmosphere. Celebrating small victories and milestones together can also enhance the sense of partnership and shared accomplishment.

Seeking Support: Sometimes, seeking external support, such as couples therapy or counseling, can be beneficial. Professional guidance can help couples navigate relationship challenges, improve communication, and develop strategies for maintaining a strong connection. Therapy can provide a safe space for addressing any issues and building a more resilient partnership.

Building a Support System

A robust support system is crucial for new parents, providing emotional, practical, and social support during the postpartum period. Building a reliable network of support helps alleviate stress, fosters wellbeing, and enhances the overall experience of parenthood.

Identifying Support Networks: Identifying and reaching out to potential sources of support is the first step in building a support system. This may include family members, friends, neighbors, and community resources. Each person or group can offer different types of support, such as practical help with baby care, emotional encouragement, or companionship.

Leveraging Family and Friends: Family and friends can be invaluable sources of support during the postpartum period. They can assist with household tasks, offer emotional support, and provide a listening ear. It's important for new parents to communicate their needs and accept help when offered. Building a support system involves actively engaging with loved ones and making the most of their willingness to assist.

Community Resources: Local community resources, such as parenting groups, support networks, and social services, can provide additional support. Parenting classes, breastfeeding support groups, and community centers often offer valuable information and a sense of connection with others in similar situations. Exploring these resources can provide practical advice, social interaction, and emotional support.

Online Support Networks: Online communities and forums can also be helpful for new parents seeking support and advice. These platforms offer opportunities to connect with other parents, share experiences, and seek guidance on various aspects of parenthood. While online support can be beneficial, it's important to balance it with in-person interactions and seek advice from trusted sources.

Balancing Independence and Support: While building a support system is essential, finding a balance between seeking help and maintaining independence is important. New parents should feel comfortable asking for help when needed but also strive to develop their own routines and strategies for managing parenthood. Balancing support with self-reliance contributes to a sense of confidence and competence.

Dealing with Social Expectations and Pressure

Social expectations and pressures can significantly impact new parents, affecting their emotional wellbeing and overall experience of parenthood. Navigating these expectations involves understanding societal norms, managing external pressures, and prioritizing personal values and needs.

Understanding Social Expectations: Societal expectations surrounding parenthood can create pressure to meet certain standards or ideals. These expectations may include notions of perfect parenting, achieving quick postpartum recovery, or balancing various roles seamlessly. Recognizing that these expectations may not reflect individual realities is the first step in managing societal pressure.

Managing External Pressures: External pressures can come from various sources, including family, friends, and social media. It's important for new parents to set boundaries and prioritize their own needs and values. Communicating openly with loved ones about their expectations and establishing realistic goals can help manage external pressures effectively.

Prioritizing Personal Values: Each family has unique values and priorities that may differ from societal norms. New parents should focus on what works best for their family and align their decisions with their values. Embracing personal preferences and making choices that reflect their own needs and goals can help mitigate the impact of social expectations.

Self-Compassion and Realism: Practicing self-compassion and maintaining realistic expectations can help manage the stress associated with societal pressures. Understanding that perfection is not attainable and acknowledging that making mistakes is part of the journey can alleviate feelings of inadequacy. Embracing imperfections and celebrating small successes contribute to a more positive outlook.

Seeking Support: If social pressures become overwhelming, seeking support from professionals or support groups can be beneficial. Counseling or therapy can provide a safe space to explore feelings and develop coping strategies. Connecting with other parents who share similar experiences can also offer validation and encouragement.

Seeking Community Support and Resources

Community support and resources play a crucial role in providing assistance, information, and connection during the postpartum period. Engaging with local and online resources can enhance the overall experience of parenthood and provide valuable support.

Exploring Local Resources: Many communities offer resources and programs designed to support new parents. These may include parenting classes, breastfeeding support groups, and family services. Exploring local resources can provide practical information, emotional support, and opportunities to connect with others in similar situations.

Accessing Healthcare Services: Healthcare providers can offer valuable support and guidance during the postpartum period. Regular check-ups, consultations with lactation consultants, and access to mental health professionals are essential components of postpartum care. Utilizing these services ensures that both physical and emotional health needs are addressed.

Utilizing Online Resources: Online platforms offer a wealth of information and support for new parents. Websites, forums, and social media groups provide access to parenting advice, peer support, and community connections. Online resources can complement local support by offering additional perspectives and information.

Connecting with Support Groups: Joining support groups can provide a sense of community and understanding. These groups, whether in-person or online, offer opportunities to share experiences, seek advice, and receive encouragement. Support groups can be especially beneficial for addressing common challenges and building a network of supportive peers.

Finding Financial and Practical Assistance: Some communities offer financial and practical assistance to new parents, such as food banks, housing support, or parenting resources. Exploring available assistance programs can help ease financial burdens and provide additional support during the postpartum period.

CHAPTER 11: RETURNING TO WORK AND DAILY LIFE

Preparing for the Transition Back to Work

Returning to work after a period of parental leave is a significant transition that requires thoughtful planning and preparation. Successfully navigating this transition involves balancing professional responsibilities with new parenting duties and ensuring a smooth reentry into the workplace.

Planning Ahead: Start preparing for your return to work well in advance. Review your company's policies on parental leave and discuss your return with your supervisor or HR department. Clarify any changes in your role or schedule and discuss how your workload will be managed upon your return. Understanding your options and setting expectations can help ease the transition.

Arranging Childcare: One of the most crucial aspects of preparing for your return to work is arranging reliable childcare. Research and explore different childcare options, such as daycare centers, in-home nannies, or family support. Visit potential providers, check references, and ensure they meet your standards for care and safety. Secure your childcare arrangements well before your return date to avoid last-minute stress.

Re-establishing a Routine: As you approach your return date, start re-establishing a routine that incorporates work and childcare. Gradually adjust your daily schedule to align with your new work hours. This may involve waking up earlier, preparing meals in advance, or practicing your commute. A smooth transition into a routine can help your family adapt more easily to the changes.

Communicating with Your Employer: Open communication with your employer is essential. Discuss any flexible work arrangements or accommodations that may be needed, such as adjusted hours, remote work options, or lactation breaks. Ensure you understand any updates or changes to workplace policies that may affect you. Clear communication helps set expectations and facilitates a supportive work environment.

Emotional Preparation: Returning to work after maternity leave can be emotionally challenging. It's normal to feel a mix of excitement, anxiety, and guilt. Acknowledge these feelings and find ways to manage them, such as talking to a trusted friend or counselor. Setting realistic goals and reminding yourself of your achievements can help build confidence as you re-enter the workforce.

Balancing Work and Motherhood

Balancing work and motherhood is a dynamic process that requires ongoing adjustment and flexibility. Finding equilibrium between professional responsibilities and parenting duties involves strategic planning, time management, and self-care.

Setting Priorities: Establishing clear priorities helps manage the demands of work and motherhood. Identify what is most important in both areas and focus on these priorities. This may involve setting boundaries at work, such as limiting overtime, and prioritizing quality time with your child. By aligning your actions with your priorities, you can better manage your responsibilities.

Creating a Support Network: Building a support network is essential for balancing work and motherhood. Rely on family, friends, and colleagues for assistance with childcare, household tasks, or emotional support. Sharing responsibilities and seeking help when needed can alleviate stress and provide a stronger support system.

Implementing Time Management Strategies: Effective time management is key to balancing work and motherhood. Create a daily or weekly schedule that incorporates work tasks, childcare, and personal time. Utilize tools such as planners, calendars, or digital apps to organize your schedule and stay on track. Allocate specific times for work, family activities, and self-care to maintain balance.

Practicing Flexibility: Flexibility is crucial when balancing work and motherhood. Be prepared to adapt your plans and expectations as needed. This may involve adjusting your work hours, seeking temporary childcare solutions, or modifying your daily routine. Embracing flexibility helps manage unexpected challenges and maintain a balanced approach to both work and family life.

Self-Care and Boundaries: Prioritizing self-care and setting boundaries are essential for maintaining balance. Make time for activities that recharge and rejuvenate you, such as exercise, hobbies, or relaxation. Set clear boundaries between work and personal time to avoid burnout and ensure you have time to focus on your family and self-care.

Childcare Options and Considerations

Choosing the right childcare option is a critical decision for working parents. Various options are available, each with its own advantages and considerations. Evaluating these options carefully helps ensure that your child receives quality care while you manage your professional responsibilities.

Types of Childcare Options: Several childcare options are available, including daycare centers, in-home nannies, family daycare, and informal care by relatives or friends. Each option has unique benefits:

- **Daycare Centers**: Daycare centers offer structured environments with trained staff and socialization opportunities for children. They may have set hours and a curriculum designed to support early development. However, they may also involve higher costs and limited flexibility.
- **In-Home Nannies**: Hiring an in-home nanny provides personalized care in the comfort of your home. Nannies can offer flexible hours and individualized attention. This option can be more expensive than other forms of childcare and may require careful vetting and background checks.
- **Family Daycare**: Family daycare is often provided in the caregiver's home. This option can offer a more intimate setting and may be less expensive than daycare centers. However, it's essential to ensure that the provider meets safety and regulatory standards.
- **Informal Care**: Relying on family members or friends for childcare can be cost-effective and provide a familiar environment for your child. However, it's important to establish clear expectations and boundaries to maintain healthy relationships and ensure consistent care.

Evaluating Quality and Safety: When selecting a childcare option, prioritize quality and safety. Visit potential providers, observe their environments, and ask about their qualifications, policies, and procedures. Ensure that the provider follows safety regulations, has appropriate certifications, and offers a supportive and nurturing environment.

Considerations for Choosing: Several factors influence the choice of childcare, including cost, location, hours, and the caregiver's approach. Consider your family's needs, budget, and preferences when making a decision. Balancing these factors helps find a solution that aligns with your work schedule and childcare requirements.

Transitioning to Childcare: Once you've selected a childcare option, plan for a smooth transition. Gradually introduce your child to their new caregiver or environment to help them adjust. Communicate openly with the caregiver about your child's needs, routines, and any concerns you may have..

Time Management and Self-Care

Effective time management and self-care are essential for balancing the demands of work and motherhood. Managing your time efficiently and taking care of yourself contribute to a healthier and more fulfilling lifestyle.

Time Management Techniques: Implementing time management techniques helps organize your daily schedule and balance work and personal responsibilities. Use tools such as planners, calendars, or digital apps to track tasks and appointments. Prioritize tasks based on urgency and importance, and break larger tasks into smaller, manageable steps.

Creating a Routine: Establishing a daily routine provides structure and predictability. Develop a schedule that includes work hours, childcare, household tasks, and personal time. Consistent routines help streamline activities and reduce stress, making it easier to manage competing demands.

Delegating Responsibilities: Delegate tasks and responsibilities to others when possible. Share household duties with your partner, family members, or colleagues. Delegating tasks helps reduce your workload and allows you to focus on essential activities and self-care.

Incorporating Self-Care: Prioritize self-care to maintain physical and emotional well-being. Allocate time for activities that rejuvenate you, such as exercise, hobbies, or relaxation. Self-care is crucial for managing stress, preventing burnout, and enhancing overall health. Make self-care a regular part of your routine, even if it's just a few minutes each day.

Setting Boundaries: Establish clear boundaries between work and personal life. Avoid bringing work home or checking emails during family time. Setting boundaries helps prevent work from encroaching on personal time and allows you to fully engage with your family and self-care activities.

Seeking Support: Don't hesitate to seek support when needed. Reach out to family, friends, or professional services for assistance with childcare, household tasks, or emotional support. Having a strong support network helps manage responsibilities and provides additional resources for coping with stress

CHAPTER 12: SPECIAL CONSIDERATIONS

Recovery After Multiple Births (Twins, Triplets, etc.)

Recovering after multiple births, such as twins or triplets, presents unique challenges and considerations compared to a single birth. The physical, emotional, and logistical aspects of postpartum recovery can be more complex and require tailored approaches to ensure a healthy recovery for both mother and babies.

Physical Recovery: The physical recovery process after multiple births can be more demanding due to the increased strain on the body during pregnancy and delivery. Mothers of multiples often experience more intense fatigue, greater physical discomfort, and longer recovery times compared to single-birth pregnancies. It is crucial to follow a comprehensive postpartum care plan, including rest, proper nutrition, and gradual return to physical activity. Monitoring for signs of complications, such as excessive bleeding or infections, is also essential.

Increased Fatigue and Stress: Managing the care of multiple newborns simultaneously can lead to significant physical and emotional fatigue. Sleep deprivation is common, and the need for constant care can exacerbate stress levels. Establishing a support system is vital; this may include enlisting help from family, friends, or professional caregivers. Prioritizing sleep and finding moments to rest and recharge are important for maintaining overall well-being.

Feeding and Nutrition: Feeding multiples can present challenges, whether breastfeeding or bottlefeeding. For breastfeeding mothers, it may be necessary to develop a feeding schedule that accommodates the needs of both babies. Techniques such as tandem nursing or using breast pumps to manage milk supply can be beneficial. For bottle-feeding, preparing and organizing feeding supplies in advance can help streamline the process.

Emotional and Psychological Support: The emotional and psychological impact of caring for multiple newborns can be profound. Feelings of overwhelm, anxiety, and even depression are common. Seeking support from a counselor, joining support groups for parents of multiples, and maintaining open communication with a partner or support network can help manage these emotional challenges.

Practical Considerations: Managing daily routines and logistics with multiple infants requires careful planning. Creating a structured schedule for feeding, sleeping, and other activities can help establish a sense of order. Investing in practical tools, such as double or triple strollers and organized baby gear, can make daily tasks more manageable. Additionally, seeking advice from other parents of multiples or professional advisors can provide valuable insights and strategies.

Postpartum Recovery for Adoptive Mothers

Postpartum recovery for adoptive mothers encompasses unique considerations and experiences compared to biological childbirth. Although the physical aspects of recovery may differ, the emotional and psychological aspects of transitioning to motherhood are similarly significant.

Emotional Transition: Adoptive mothers may experience a range of emotions as they transition into their new role. This can include joy, anxiety, and feelings of inadequacy. It is important for adoptive mothers to recognize and address these emotions, seeking support from therapists, support groups, or friends. Understanding that these feelings are normal and seeking professional guidance can aid in navigating this transition.

Bonding with the Baby: Building a bond with an adopted child can be a deeply fulfilling experience, but it may take time. Adoptive mothers can foster bonding through activities such as skin-to-skin contact, responsive caregiving, and spending quality time together. Participating in activities that promote attachment, such as reading, singing, and physical affection, can strengthen the emotional connection with the baby.

Managing Expectations: Adoptive mothers may face societal or self-imposed expectations regarding their parenting journey. It is important to manage these expectations and focus on the unique relationship being built with the adopted child. Setting realistic goals and celebrating small milestones can help in adjusting to the new role and finding satisfaction in the parenting experience.

Support Networks: Building a support network is crucial for adoptive mothers. This may involve connecting with other adoptive parents, joining support groups, or seeking guidance from professionals specializing in adoption. Sharing experiences, receiving advice, and finding reassurance from others who have undergone similar experiences can provide valuable support and perspective.

Self-Care and Well-Being: Taking care of oneself is essential for adoptive mothers to ensure overall wellbeing. This includes managing stress, maintaining physical health, and finding time for self-care. Balancing the demands of parenting with self-care practices, such as regular exercise, healthy eating, and relaxation, contributes to a positive postpartum experience.

Recovering After Miscarriage or Stillbirth

Recovering from a miscarriage or stillbirth is an emotionally and physically challenging experience. The process of healing involves addressing both the grief and physical aspects of recovery, while also seeking support and finding ways to cope with the loss.

Emotional Healing: The emotional impact of miscarriage or stillbirth can be profound and multifaceted. Feelings of grief, sadness, anger, and confusion are common. It is important to allow oneself to grieve and seek support from counselors, support groups, or trusted friends and family. Engaging in open conversations about the loss and finding ways to honor the memory of the baby can aid in the healing process.

Physical Recovery: Physically recovering from a miscarriage or stillbirth involves monitoring for any medical issues and following healthcare provider recommendations. This may include managing bleeding, pain, or any complications that arise. It is essential to attend follow-up appointments to ensure proper recovery and address any health concerns.

Managing Expectations: The experience of miscarriage or stillbirth may come with societal or selfimposed expectations regarding grief and recovery. It is important to acknowledge that healing is a personal journey and may take time. Setting realistic expectations for oneself and seeking professional guidance when needed can help manage this aspect of recovery.

Support Systems: Building a strong support system is crucial for coping with the loss. Connecting with others who have experienced similar losses, Joining support groups, and seeking professional counseling can provide valuable comfort and understanding. Family and friends can also play a supportive role in providing empathy and assistance during the recovery process.

Self-Care and Healing: Prioritizing self-care is important for both emotional and physical healing. Engaging in activities that promote relaxation and well-being, such as gentle exercise, meditation, or creative outlets, can support the recovery process. It is also essential to be patient with oneself and allow time for healing.

CHAPTER 13: LONG-TERM HEALTH AND WELLBEING

Maintaining Physical Health

Maintaining physical health in the long term after childbirth involves a holistic approach that includes a balanced diet, regular exercise, sufficient sleep, and consistent medical check-ups. The postpartum period doesn't end when the baby turns one; instead, it marks the beginning of a lifelong journey of health and wellness that needs careful nurturing.

Balanced Diet: Nutrition plays a crucial role in maintaining physical health. Postpartum, a mother's body requires nutrients to recover, especially if she is breastfeeding. A balanced diet rich in whole foods, including fruits, vegetables, lean proteins, whole grains, and healthy fats, is essential. Adequate calcium and iron intake is particularly important for bone health and to replenish iron stores depleted during childbirth. Staying hydrated is equally vital, as it aids digestion, helps with milk production, and supports overall bodily functions.

Regular Exercise: Incorporating regular physical activity into daily routines can improve cardiovascular health, boost mood, and help maintain a healthy weight. However, exercise should be approached gradually, especially if there were complications during delivery or if a cesarean section was performed. Low-impact activities like walking, swimming, and yoga are excellent starting points. As strength and stamina improve, higher intensity workouts can be incorporated. It's essential to listen to the body and consult with a healthcare provider before starting any new exercise regimen.

Sleep and Rest: While the early postpartum period is often associated with sleep deprivation, establishing healthy sleep habits is crucial for long-term well-being. Good sleep hygiene, such as maintaining a consistent sleep schedule and creating a restful environment, can significantly impact physical and mental health. Naps can be beneficial, particularly when nighttime sleep is interrupted by childcare responsibilities.

Medical Check-ups: Regular medical check-ups are vital for monitoring recovery and overall health. These appointments provide an opportunity to address any ongoing or new concerns, such as hormonal imbalances, chronic fatigue, or lingering pain. Regular screenings for conditions like diabetes, hypertension, and thyroid disorders are also important, as pregnancy can increase the risk of these conditions.

Managing Chronic Conditions: If chronic conditions existed before or developed during pregnancy, managing them effectively is crucial. Conditions like gestational diabetes or pregnancy-induced hypertension require ongoing monitoring and lifestyle adjustments to prevent them from progressing to more severe health issues.

Incorporating Healthy Habits: Developing and maintaining healthy habits is key to long-term physical health. This includes mindful eating, staying active, managing stress, and avoiding harmful substances like tobacco and excessive alcohol. Integrating these habits into daily life can provide lasting benefits and improve overall quality of life.

Maintaining physical health postpartum is a dynamic and ongoing process. By focusing on a balanced diet, regular exercise, sufficient sleep, and consistent medical care, mothers can support their physical health and enjoy a vibrant and fulfilling life.

Mental Health Maintenance

Maintaining mental health after the postpartum period is an ongoing journey that requires attention and care. The transition to motherhood, while joyous, can bring about significant changes and challenges that impact mental well-being. Proactive strategies and supportive resources are crucial for sustaining mental health in the long term.

Understanding the Impact: The postpartum period can be marked by a range of emotions, from happiness and fulfillment to anxiety and depression. It's important to recognize that these feelings can persist beyond the immediate postpartum phase. Hormonal changes, sleep deprivation, and the stress of adapting to new roles can all contribute to mental health challenges. Acknowledging these experiences and understanding that they are normal can be the first step towards maintaining mental health.

Building a Support System: A strong support system is vital for mental well-being. This can include partners, family members, friends, and healthcare professionals. Open communication with these individuals can provide emotional support, practical assistance, and reassurance. Support groups, whether in-person or online, can also offer a sense of community and understanding from those experiencing similar challenges.

Professional Help: Seeking professional help, such as therapy or counseling, is a valuable tool for maintaining mental health. Therapists can provide a safe space to explore emotions, develop coping strategies, and address specific concerns like anxiety, depression, or post-traumatic stress related to childbirth. Cognitive-behavioral therapy (CBT), mindfulness practices, and other therapeutic approaches can be particularly beneficial.

Self-Care Practices: Self-care is an essential component of mental health maintenance. This involves setting aside time for activities that bring joy and relaxation, such as reading, hobbies, or spending time outdoors. Mindfulness practices, such as meditation and deep breathing exercises, can help reduce stress and improve emotional regulation. It's also important to prioritize self-compassion, allowing oneself to experience a full range of emotions without judgment.

Managing Expectations: Adjusting expectations is crucial for mental health. The pressures of modern motherhood, including societal expectations and self-imposed standards, can be overwhelming. It's important to set realistic goals, acknowledge limitations, and celebrate small victories. Recognizing that it's okay to ask for help and that not everything will be perfect can relieve undue pressure and improve overall well-being.

Balancing Responsibilities: Finding a balance between parenting duties, work, and personal life is key to sustaining mental health. Time management skills, delegating tasks, and setting boundaries can help prevent burnout. It's also beneficial to plan for downtime and rest, ensuring that the demands of motherhood do not overshadow personal needs and well-being.

Monitoring and Adapting: Mental health is not static, and it's important to regularly assess and adapt strategies as needed. Life changes, such as returning to work or transitioning through different stages of child development, can bring new challenges. Continuously monitoring one's mental state and being open to adjusting coping strategies can help maintain balance and resilience.

Maintaining mental health postpartum is a dynamic and evolving process. By building a strong support system, seeking professional help, practicing self-care, managing expectations, and finding balance, mothers can foster long-term mental well-being and enjoy a fulfilling motherhood experience.

Planning for Future Pregnancies

Planning for future pregnancies involves a thoughtful and proactive approach to ensure the health and well-being of both the mother and potential future children. Whether immediately after a previous birth or several years later, considering factors like physical health, mental readiness, and lifestyle adjustments is crucial.

Assessing Physical Health: Before planning another pregnancy, it's important to assess overall physical health. This includes consulting with a healthcare provider to review any medical conditions, previous pregnancy complications, and overall fitness. Conditions such as diabetes, hypertension, or thyroid disorders should be managed effectively before conceiving. If a cesarean section was performed, discussing the recommended time for the uterus to heal and considering the safest delivery options for future pregnancies is crucial.

Nutritional Preparedness: Adequate nutrition plays a vital role in preparing for a healthy pregnancy. Ensuring a balanced diet rich in essential nutrients like folic acid, iron, calcium, and vitamin D is important for the health of both the mother and the developing fetus. Folic acid is particularly crucial as it helps prevent neural tube defects in the early stages of pregnancy. For women planning to conceive, starting a prenatal vitamin regimen before pregnancy can provide essential nutrients and support optimal health.

Mental and Emotional Readiness: Mental and emotional readiness is just as important as physical health. Reflecting on the experience of the previous postpartum period and addressing any lingering mental health issues, such as postpartum depression or anxiety, is crucial. Couples should communicate openly about their readiness and any concerns, ensuring that both partners are on the same page regarding expanding their family. Seeking counseling or therapy can be beneficial for addressing any unresolved emotional challenges or stressors.

Timing and Spacing: The timing and spacing of pregnancies can significantly impact maternal and child health. Research suggests that a minimum interpregnancy interval of 18 to 24 months reduces the risk of complications like preterm birth and low birth weight. However, the optimal timing may vary based on individual health circumstances and personal preferences. Discussing the ideal timing with a healthcare provider can help in making an informed decision.

Lifestyle Adjustments: Preparing for another pregnancy may require lifestyle adjustments, such as quitting smoking, reducing alcohol intake, and achieving a healthy weight. Regular physical activity can improve cardiovascular health, reduce stress, and prepare the body for the physical demands of pregnancy. Additionally, managing stress through mindfulness practices, hobbies, or other relaxation techniques can create a healthier environment for conception and pregnancy.

Financial and Logistical Considerations: Planning for future pregnancies also involves considering financial and logistical aspects. Assessing the family's financial situation, planning for potential healthcare costs, and ensuring adequate health insurance coverage are important steps. Additionally, considering the need for extra space, childcare arrangements, and potential changes in work schedules can help ease the transition and reduce stress.

Monitoring and Preparing: Finally, ongoing monitoring and preparation are essential. Regular health check-ups, staying informed about pregnancy-related health issues, and maintaining open communication with healthcare providers can help address any emerging concerns and ensure a healthy pregnancy. Planning for future pregnancies involves a comprehensive approach that considers physical health, mental and emotional readiness, timing, lifestyle adjustments, and practical considerations. By taking these factors into account and seeking professional guidance, couples can optimize their chances for a healthy and fulfilling pregnancy experience.

Long-Term Pelvic Health

Long-term pelvic health is a critical aspect of overall well-being for women, particularly following childbirth. The pelvic floor muscles play a key role in supporting the bladder, bowel, and uterus, as well as in maintaining continence and sexual function. Ensuring the health and strength of these muscles postpartum is essential for preventing long-term complications and enhancing quality of life.

Pelvic Floor Rehabilitation: Pregnancy and childbirth, especially vaginal delivery, can weaken the pelvic floor muscles. This weakening can lead to issues such as urinary incontinence, pelvic organ pro-lapse, and reduced sexual sensation. Pelvic floor rehabilitation involves exercises designed to strengthen these muscles and restore their function. Kegel exercises are a well-known and effective method for pelvic floor strengthening. Regularly practicing these exercises can improve muscle tone, enhance bladder control, and reduce the risk of prolapse.

Professional Guidance: Seeking professional guidance from a pelvic floor physical therapist can be invaluable. These specialists can provide tailored exercise programs, manual therapies, and education to help women regain pelvic floor strength and function. They can also address specific issues such as pain during intercourse, scar tissue management after a cesarean section or episiotomy, and strategies for preventing prolapse.

Maintaining a Healthy Weight: Maintaining a healthy weight is important for pelvic health. Excess weight can place additional strain on the pelvic floor muscles, exacerbating issues like incontinence and prolapse. A balanced diet and regular physical activity can help achieve and maintain a healthy weight, reducing the load on the pelvic floor and improving overall health.

Avoiding Strain: Avoiding unnecessary strain on the pelvic floor is crucial. Activities that increase abdominal pressure, such as heavy lifting, high-impact exercises, and chronic coughing, can weaken the pelvic floor over time. Proper lifting techniques, managing chronic coughs or allergies, and choosing lowimpact exercises can help protect the pelvic floor.

Addressing Constipation: Chronic constipation can lead to straining during bowel movements, which can weaken the pelvic floor muscles. Managing constipation through a diet rich in fiber, adequate hydration, and, if necessary, the use of stool softeners can prevent straining and protect pelvic health. Regular bowel habits and proper positioning during defecation (such as using a footstool to elevate the feet) can also reduce strain.

Hormonal Considerations: Hormonal changes, particularly during menopause, can affect pelvic health. The decline in estrogen levels can lead to thinning and weakening of the vaginal and urethral tissues, increasing the risk of incontinence and pelvic organ prolapse. Hormone replacement therapy (HRT) or local estrogen treatments may be recommended for some women to maintain tissue health and function.

Regular Check-ups: Regular pelvic exams and screenings are essential for monitoring pelvic health. These check-ups can help detect early signs of prolapse, incontinence, or other issues, allowing for timely intervention. Women should discuss any pelvic floor concerns with their healthcare provider, including symptoms like urinary leakage, pelvic pressure, or discomfort.

Lifestyle Modifications: Long-term pelvic health can be supported by making lifestyle modifications, such as quitting smoking, which can reduce the risk of chronic coughing, and avoiding excessive caffeine and alcohol, which can irritate the bladder. Staying informed about pelvic health and being proactive in seeking care can empower women to maintain their pelvic health and prevent complications.

In conclusion, long-term pelvic health requires a proactive and informed approach. Through pelvic floor exercises, professional guidance, maintaining a healthy weight, avoiding strain, managing constipation, addressing hormonal changes, and regular check-ups, women can protect and enhance their pelvic health, ensuring a higher quality of life and overall well-being.

Preventive Health Screenings

Preventive health screenings are an essential component of long-term health and well-being, especially for women who have gone through childbirth. These screenings are designed to detect potential health issues early, allowing for timely intervention and treatment. Regular check-ups and appropriate screenings can help prevent serious health conditions and maintain overall health.

Breast Cancer Screening: One of the most important preventive health screenings for women is breast cancer screening. Mammograms are recommended starting at age 40 or earlier for those with a family history or other risk factors. Self-examinations and clinical breast exams are also important for early detection. Breastfeeding can slightly reduce the risk of breast cancer, but regular screening remains crucial for all women.

Cervical Cancer Screening: Cervical cancer screening through Pap smears and HPV testing is vital for detecting precancerous changes in the cervix. Women should begin screening at age 21 and continue at regular intervals as recommended by their healthcare provider. The frequency of screenings may vary based on age, health history, and test results. Vaccination against HPV can also help prevent cervical cancer.

Bone Density Testing: Bone density testing, or DEXA scans, is important for assessing the risk of osteoporosis, especially in women who have experienced pregnancy-related bone loss or have other risk factors like a family history of osteoporosis or long-term steroid use. Women should discuss the appropriate timing for this screening with their healthcare provider, especially as they approach menopause.

Cardiovascular Health Screening: Pregnancy can sometimes reveal or exacerbate underlying cardiovascular conditions. Therefore, monitoring cardiovascular health postpartum is crucial. Screenings for blood pressure, cholesterol levels, and blood sugar are important for detecting hypertension, hyperlipidemia, and diabetes, which are risk factors for heart disease. Maintaining a heart-healthy lifestyle with a balanced diet, regular exercise, and stress management is also essential.

Diabetes Screening: Women who had gestational diabetes during pregnancy are at an increased risk of developing type 2 diabetes later in life. It is recommended that these women undergo regular screening for diabetes, starting at six to 12 weeks postpartum and continuing every one to three years. Early detection allows for lifestyle modifications and, if necessary, medication to manage blood sugar levels.

Thyroid Function Testing: Postpartum thyroiditis is a condition that can affect thyroid function after childbirth. Symptoms can include fatigue, weight changes, and mood swings, which can easily be mistaken for typical postpartum experiences. Thyroid function tests, including TSH and T4 levels, can help diagnose thyroid disorders, ensuring appropriate treatment and management.

Mental Health Screenings: Mental health is a crucial aspect of overall well-being. Screening for conditions like depression and anxiety, particularly postpartum depression, should be a routine part of postpartum care. Questionnaires and discussions with healthcare providers can help identify symptoms early, allowing for timely intervention and support.

Pelvic Health Assessments: As part of preventive care, regular pelvic exams are important for assessing pelvic floor health, detecting issues like pelvic organ prolapse, and monitoring for conditions like uterine fibroids or ovarian cysts. Women should discuss any symptoms, such as pelvic pain or changes in menstrual cycles, with their healthcare provider.

Skin Cancer Screening: Skin changes during pregnancy, including increased pigmentation and the appearance of moles, can sometimes be concerning. Regular skin checks and screenings for skin cancer, especially for those with a family history or high exposure to UV radiation, are important for early detection and treatment.

Vaccinations: Keeping up to date with vaccinations, such as the flu shot, Tdap (tetanus, diphtheria, and pertussis), and the COVID-19 vaccine, is crucial for protecting both maternal and child health. Women should consult with their healthcare provider about necessary vaccinations, especially when planning future pregnancies.

CONCLUSION

The postpartum period is a multifaceted journey marked by profound physical, emotional, and practical changes. Understanding and addressing the diverse aspects of postpartum recovery are crucial for ensuring a positive and healthy transition into motherhood. This includes navigating the immediate postpartum period, managing physical recovery, and addressing the emotional and mental health challenges that arise. Each experience is unique, shaped by individual circumstances, cultural backgrounds, and personal needs.

Physical Recovery: The physical demands of postpartum recovery vary depending on the type of delivery and any complications that may have occurred. Healing after vaginal delivery or cesarean section requires tailored care, while managing pain, postpartum bleeding, and swelling are essential aspects of recovery. Special considerations, such as recovering from multiple births or addressing unique challenges like postpartum hemorrhage, highlight the need for personalized care and support.

Emotional and Mental Health: The emotional landscape of the postpartum period is complex, with experiences ranging from the baby blues to more severe conditions like postpartum depression and anxiety. Building a robust support system, seeking therapy, and engaging in self-care practices are critical for maintaining mental health. Partners and family play a vital role in providing emotional support and understanding during this transformative time.

Nutrition and Hydration: Proper nutrition and hydration are fundamental to postpartum recovery. Meeting nutritional needs, addressing special dietary considerations, and ensuring adequate hydration contribute to overall health and well-being. For breastfeeding mothers, maintaining a balanced diet and considering supplements can support both maternal and infant health.

Breastfeeding and Lactation: Successfully navigating breastfeeding and lactation involves overcoming common challenges, understanding the benefits, and learning effective pumping and storing techniques. Weaning and transitioning from breastfeeding are also important stages that require thoughtful planning and support.

Physical Fitness and Exercise: Reintroducing physical activity into your routine requires careful consideration. Safe postpartum exercises, rebuilding core strength, and strengthening the pelvic floor are essential components of a balanced fitness approach. Incorporating practices such as yoga and mindfulness can further enhance physical and emotional well-being.

Body Image and Self-Esteem: Postpartum body image and self-esteem often undergo significant changes. Navigating these changes, building a positive body image, and finding comfort in fashion choices can help foster a sense of confidence and self-worth. Reconnecting with a partner intimately also plays a role in maintaining a healthy relationship and self-esteem.

Sleep and Rest: Managing postpartum sleep deprivation involves developing strategies for better sleep and rest. Napping, managing nighttime feedings, and prioritizing rest are key to maintaining overall health and coping with the demands of caring for a newborn.

Postpartum Complications: Recognizing and managing postpartum complications, such as infections, hemorrhage, and blood clots, is critical for ensuring a safe recovery. Being aware of potential complications and seeking timely medical intervention can help address any issues that arise.

Postpartum Relationships and Social Support: Adjusting to parenthood and strengthening relationships with partners and support networks are essential for a positive postpartum experience. Building a support system, managing social expectations, and seeking community resources contribute to a balanced and supportive environment.

Returning to Work and Daily Life: Transitioning back to work and managing daily life requires careful preparation and time management. Balancing professional responsibilities with motherhood, exploring childcare options, and prioritizing self-care are key to navigating this transition successfully.

Special Considerations: Addressing special considerations, such as recovery after multiple births, postpartum recovery for adoptive mothers, and coping with miscarriage or stillbirth, underscores the need for individualized and compassionate care. Cultural and societal differences also play a significant role in shaping postpartum experiences and care.

In conclusion, the postpartum period is a time of significant change and adaptation. By addressing the diverse aspects of postpartum recovery, from physical healing and emotional support to practical considerations and special circumstances, individuals can navigate this journey with greater confidence and well-being. Support from healthcare providers, family, and community resources plays a vital role in fostering a positive postpartum experience and ensuring a healthy transition into motherhood.